HEALING
CONNECTIONS

HEALING CONNECTIONS

Bridging Body and Mind

MIRIAM SPERBER

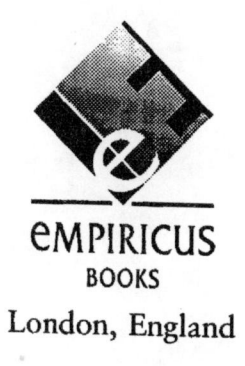

eMPIRICUS
BOOKS
London, England

First published in Great Britain 1999
by Empiricus Books,
76 Great Titchfield Street,
London W1P 7AF

www.januspublishing.co.uk

Copyright © 1999 by Miriam Sperber
The author has asserted her moral rights

A CIP catalogue record for this book
is available from the British Library.

ISBN: 1 902 835 04 2

Phototypeset in 11.5 on 13.5 Sabon
by Keyboard Services, Luton, Beds

Cover design by Peter Clarke

Printed and bound in Great Britain

To the memory of my spiritual mentor,
Joseph Gikatilla

*A mind not to be changed by place or time.
The mind is its own place, and in itself
Can make a Heaven of Hell, a Hell of Heaven.*

John Milton, *Paradise Lost*

Contents

Acknowledgements ix
Preface xi
Introduction xvii

PART I: THE HUMAN HOLOGRAM — 1
1 The Brain's Playing Fields — 3
2 An Infinite Sphere — 21
3 Acting As Man: the Machine Barrier — 31
4 Soul Searching — 39

PART II: MESSAGES FROM THE PAST — 49
1 The Rod and the Fire — 51
2 Healing Rivers — 62
3 The Giant of Kos — 76
4 In Tune with Eternity — 85

Healing Connections

PART III: A MIND OF OUR OWN	91
1 Mind Bridges: Scientific versus Folk Psychology	93
2 Keeping the Faith – Spirituality and Healing	101
3 Acting on Instinct and the Twists of Reason	107
Bibliography	117

Preface

On recent scientific evidence supporting the existence of a highly significant mind–body interaction in health and disease statuses

The development in recent years of alternative therapeutic techniques has inevitably resulted in a certain degree of confusion among the general public, which is clearly attracted towards the new practices, but still requires conventional medical care in instances of serious health impairment.

The academic medical establishment has invested a great deal of effort in research studies designed to verify the efficiency of certain supplementary therapeutic methods. These have been directed especially towards the demonstration of the regulatory mechanisms originating in the human brain, influencing on one hand the appearance of diseases and, on the other, recovery from them. A most comprehensive range of illnesses and techniques has been investigated, from the study of breathing and relaxation instruction in myocardial infarction patients, to aromatherapy in the treatment of chronic pain and the effects of positive imagery in the process of healing, to the influence of the emotional status of an individual on the development of migraine or respiratory symptoms, and many others.

Of great value is the ability of these studies to make a connection between the concepts relating to the physiological function of the human body, developed by illustrious medical precursors, and modern ideas. The Department of Psychology at the University of North Carolina at Charlotte, has dedicated a paper in the *Journal of Integrative Physiological & Behavioural Science* (April–June, 1997) to the renowned Russian scientist IP Pavlov's ideas concerning the mind–body problem. The concept of emotions and their influence on the body is reviewed within the great physiologist's theory of higher nervous activity.

In the same line of ideas, at the Vrije Universiteit in Amsterdam, the Department of Psychiatry has checked the concepts of 'mind' and 'body' as they are reflected in disease symptoms. These concepts have been found to be of very early origins and, while certainly supporting more 'ancient' illnesses, prove to be active in contemporary disorders that involve several body systems, and are sometimes of unclear origin, such as myalgic encephalomyelitis or the hypersensitivity syndrome.

The highly respected Harvard Medical School in Boston, US has devoted as well a great deal of attention to how 'mind–body medicine' is becoming mainstream. In an article published in May 1997 in *Hospital Practice*, the importance has been underlined of the benefits resulting from being able to control vital aspects of the body metabolism voluntarily and of making an effort to understand the mechanisms at the base of such control. At the same time, we find that the heart of contemporary research in this area is the identification of the best 'mind–body fitness programmes', i.e. making the general public familiar with the most valuable ways to improve and activate the mind–body connection, and encouraging prospects for primary and secondary disease prevention.

The main concern remains the long-term adherence of patients to health-promotion programmes. At the San Diego Cardiac Centre Medical Group in California, a lipid-disorders training programme has been introduced that combines mind–body exercise with existing health promotion and cardiac-rehabilitation services. 'Mind–body exercise' is a method of coupling muscular activity with an internally directed focus, so that the participant produces a temporary self-contemplative mental state. This internal focus is in contrast to conventional body-centred aerobic and muscular-fitness exercise in which there is little or no mindful component. Exercise programmes such as yoga and tai chi are mentioned as excellent means of combining physical and mental stimulation.

These findings support the data obtained in the newly developed field of psychoneuroimmunology, which shows that there is serious reason to take into consideration the existence of 'psychologically induced immunoenhancement'. The worldwide interest in the subject is exemplified by a study made in Munich, Germany at the Ludwig-Maximilians-Universitat in 1998, dealing with the interactions between the immune system and the psyche and demonstrating that distress-reducing techniques such as progressive relaxation training, imagery, experimentally induced positive mood-states and laughter all seem to enhance various aspects of immune functions.

When attempting to help patients suffering from chronic illnesses, the Department of Psychology and Social Behaviour at the University of California, Irvine has found that a stress-reduction programme based on training in mindfulness meditation has shown evidence of: 1 significant reduction in the overall psychological symptoms; 2 increase in the overall sense of control in the patients' lives; 3 higher scores on a measure of spiritual experiences. In general, the great diversity of human activities covered by these studies, and the variety of disease entities studied can be easily recognised when surveying some of the published titles: *Cardiorespiratory effects of breathing and relaxation instruction in myocardial infarction patients* (Kennemer Hospital, Harlem, The Netherlands, 1998); *Massage therapy effects* (University of Miami School of Medicine, 1998); *Essential oils and aromatherapy: their modern role in healing* (School of Applied Sciences, South Bank University, London, UK, 1997); *Treatment of menopausal symptoms with applied relaxation* (University Hospital, Linköping, Sweden); *Religion and healing. Cultivating a respectful ambivalence* (University of North Carolina at Chapel Hill, USA, 1998) and many others.

Based on the above, it becomes more and more evident that contemporary medicine feels that it is high time to allocate effort and financial support to the study of those age-long complementary therapeutic techniques that are able to support successfully modern pharmacological products and interventional therapies in the fight against disease. The 'healthy avenues of the mind' are complex and difficult to uncover. None the less, it seems of supreme importance that mankind continues to inquire into the mind, body, health and disease issues, to identify what we know, and what we should do about them. As a medical article published in the *Journal of American Association (JAMA)* in February 1998 stated, it becomes obvious that 'healing is more than clowning around'.

Preface

Even if numerous aspects of the intricate paths connecting mental powers to body functioning are still to be explained, scientific studies of recent years have succeeded in creating a more integrative view, in which the duality of mental and physical is replaced by the concept of an organic and psychological unity. The result is an increasingly holistic approach to medical practices, expected to increase humanity's ability to optimise physical functioning in times of health or disease. 'Mind matters' is the convincing message and, in this context, the ancient idealistic pursuit of a 'healthy mind in a healthy body' appears to be more relevant than ever.

Introduction – The Realm of the Possible

The mind is not a vessel to be filled, but a fire to be kindled.

Plutarch, *Bioi Paralleloi* (*Parallel Lives*)

The afternoon sun was illuminating my office as she stood in the centre of the room, smiling: 'Remember when they said I would never walk again?' the young woman said.

My patient looked radiant and it was indeed difficult to believe that this was the same person who several months ago was lying helplessly in a hospital bed. Being a young physician at the time, I asked myself again and again: what makes the difference? What decides in favour of one patient recovering faster than another? Why do several patients, suffering from the same disease and receiving the same treatment, react differently?

One answer is provided, of course, by the natural constitution of each organism, the state of its immune system and various other factors, including age, sex, profession and previous illnesses. I had, however, a very strong feeling that there was much more to it than that.

During my studies in medical school, the curriculum included very little information on the existence of causes, other than organic, for the origin of human diseases, and only a minimal insight into the influence exerted by the psychological makeup of an individual on his or her well-being. It was therefore with a sense of breaking new ground that, in an attempt to answer the above questions, I came to the conclusion: 'It is all in the mind.'

Undoubtedly, in view of the recent disenchantment with classical therapeutic techniques and the increased public interest in a holistic approach to medicine, this statement appears rather clichéd. The issue is, however, much more complicated than it seems. A great discrepancy can be usually found in the attitudes and opinions expressed concerning our mental and emotional capabilities, depending on the specific angle of observation. While scientific research has greatly advanced our understanding of the anatomical structure and physiological functioning of the human brain, much remains to be done in the realm of neurological investigation.

'The brain works like a computer.' As the following chapters will show, this succinct contemporary generalisation does not answer all current queries. What are the specialised areas in the brain controlling body and psychological functions? What are intelligence, willpower, creativity and intuition, and how can they be associated with specific neurological structures? What are the pathways of mental activity in illness and health? Despite the intensive exploration of the subject, the fascinating maze of neural synapses jealously preserves its secrets.

Introduction

Matters are further complicated by the various spiritual outlooks on mental capabilities and human life in general. Viewed as an inherent component of an endless natural chain, our existence on this planet is considered by many to be a voluntary and necessary act, directed and continuously influenced by a superior divine power. There have been many attempts to define what appears to be beyond our grasp, in particular the issue of what separates human beings from the animal kingdom. What makes people capable of reasoning, dreaming, transmitting knowledge, suffering and comprehending in such a unique and unmistakable manner?

With numerous authors attempting to develop a philosophical approach to the subject of human intelligence, it is obvious that illustrious precursors such as Sigmund Freud and CG Jung, or contemporary thinkers such as David Rosenthal or Roger Penrose, have added valuable dimensions to our search for the hidden and profound human essence without, however, closing all the chapters. Human skills, aspirations, problems and concerns, extraordinary and unequalled as they are, remain a baffling element in comparison with *l'homme machine*, the 'man acting as a machine' described so well by the French and, in general, as demonstrated by recent works with any artificial intelligence, however advanced.

The idea for the present book came to me as a natural result of pondering for many years on the above issues. I felt that the material could satisfy both a reader's interest in comprehending the way the human mind works, and his or her desire to learn the most appropriate means of utilising the tremendous positive energies stored in the human psyche. Moreover, modern health practitioners could certainly benefit from the study of the healing traditions of our ancestors, in different epochs and cultures around the globe, where the pursuit for medical cures and human happiness means understanding the disease sufferer in a profound and all-embracing manner, including physical and psychological aspects.

The classical medical doctrines of Hippocrates and Galen preclude modern-day dilemmas related to how medicine can solve the issues raised by the increasing stresses and strains of daily life. Modern clinical experience continues to support the teachings of these medical luminaries, by emphasising the value of positive thinking, dedicated personal care, and an intuitive approach in medical decision making. In addition, the importance is underlined of the patient's personal contribution in the healing process, particularly his or her constructive attitude towards therapy.

In an era where new technological devices are being developed continuously, where 'miracle' drugs permit organ transplants, and genetic engineering becomes part of daily routine, people are still confronted by their inability to cope with an increasing number of psychosomatic disorders. The achieved longevity of mankind today, far from representing the promised golden age, has only added more patients to the list of those unable to handle the inescapable passage of time. Additionally, and not surprisingly, the formative and active years are still the human stages when support and advice are most needed.

I trust that by combining and exhibiting several updated and intriguing viewpoints on the subject of medicine and the mind, the present book will carry a message of hope for achieving success and the best of health during one's lifetime. Our mind, our friend and counsellor, is there to guide us. The ray of light contained in it, connecting the entire hierarchy of living things in the universe, provides all the necessary resources for a supply of natural wellness, resilience in the face of adversity, a disposition to take a bright, hopeful view of things, and an endless love of life.

PART I

THE HUMAN HOLOGRAM

Chapter 1

The Brain's Playing Fields

> *Water is H_2O, hydrogen two parts, oxygen one, but there is also a third thing, that makes it water and nobody knows what that is.*
>
> DH Lawrence, *Pansies, The Third Thing*

Undoubtedly one of the most intriguing and complex objects in the universe, the human brain is an organ, the basic structure of which is not too difficult to comprehend. In fact, our brain's anatomical components have long been recognised in different representatives of the animal kingdom, in a wide variety of developmental stages. This has prompted the idea of the human brain being the result of a long evolutionary process, at the end of which Man occupies a highly enviable place, that of the most 'intelligent' creature. The latter means that a special capability exists to perceive, act, feel, learn and remember, unmistakably specific to a human being and not found in other living species.

A detailed review of the brain's anatomy is beyond the scope of this book. I will, however, mention some of the most relevant constituents, as most of our present understanding of the brain's activity is based on the study of the relationship of a specific function (perception, thought or movement), to a particular brain region, with its anatomical and physiological characteristics.

As pictured in the figure below, the main components of the human central nervous system are the cerebrum, the cerebellum, the brain stem and the spinal cord. A series of structures

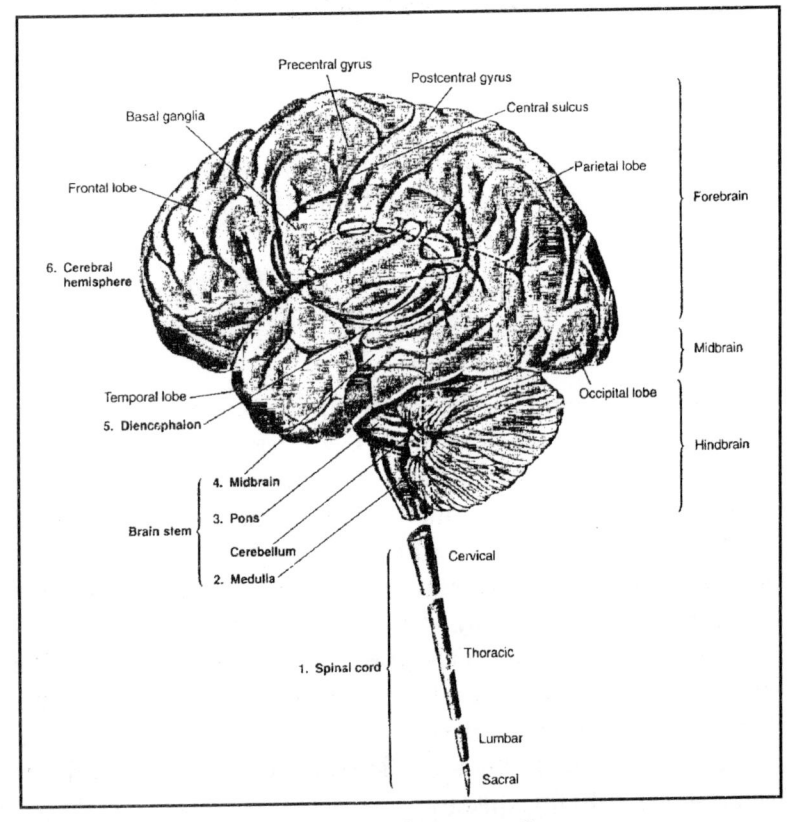

The Human Central Nervous System

is situated between the cerebrum and the brain stem, most importantly the thalamus, which is a sensory integration centre connected to many areas of the brain, and the hypothalamus, which is in charge of the pivotal autonomic nervous system regulating the endocrine glands, the smooth muscles and the heart.

While the brain stem supervises such vital functions as breathing and digestion, the spinal cord controls the movements of the limbs and the trunk, and also receives sensory information from the skin, joints and muscles in these regions. Aside from the two cerebral hemispheres, higher mental and emotional activities require the participation of a great number of brain elements, some of them known for a different primary function. A good example is the spinal cord, which additionally to its control over motor functions also adjusts levels of arousal and awareness. Similarly, the olfactory system controls the sense of smelland plays a role in forming emotions, as observed in animals who tend to sniffle each other, or in the human well-known preoccupation with perfume.

The cerebral hemispheres are covered by a largely convoluted cortex, divided according to the overlying cranial bones, in four lobes each: frontal, parietal, temporal and occipital. Some of the most important centres mastering movement, sight and hearing are located in the frontal, occipital and temporal regions, respectively. Large portions of cortex named 'association areas', situated outside these regions, are used for more complex brain functions, such as perception and motivation.

A 'motivational system' supervises the intricate cooperation between all the enumerated neural centres. A very important constituent, this system seems to have the extraordinary ability of inducing particular actions, such as drinking or smiling, and at the same time coordinating, fusing and refining various motor and autonomic reactions that compose a wide range of human activities.

A dancer's performance, for example, will be based on an elaborate mixture of motor movements and sensory perceptions. The motivational or limbic system will be the one that decides on the final completion and quality of the act, as it implies the participation of involuntary features (such as sweating or an increased heart beat), together with awareness of the surroundings, skill, and mainly mental concentration and excitement.

The French surgeon and anthropologist Paul Broca, who made extensive comparative studies of crania and brains in various human races, is credited with the discovery of the centre of articulate speech, located in the anterior part of the left brain, a place now named Broca's area. A revolutionary finding, it provided the first anatomical proof for a functional localisation in the brain. Broca is also the one who, in 1878, introduced the concept of a limbic system, later developed to describe a special neural circuit in the region surrounding the upper brain stem. This area is considered to represent the most ancient cortex on the evolutionary scale, and is known to play a critical role in the expression of emotions and the way they reach consciousness and thought.

Activity at the cellular level in the central nervous system involves basic functional units named neurons, which transmit almost instantaneous information from one part of the body to the other. Each neuron is composed of a cell body containing a nucleus and tiny filaments called dendrites, which extend from the cellular body and are specialised in receiving electrical signals from dendrites of other nerve cells.

Additionally, there is a long extension named the axon, through which a nervous impulse is carried away from the cell body to the dendrites of the neighbouring nerve. The point of contact between the two is known as a synapse, where several chemical products named neurotransmitters transmit neural impulses.

It is a very difficult task to discuss any type of mental activity based on this extremely concise presentation of brain anatomy. The reason for it is not difficult to comprehend. Some 100 billion neurons compose the average human brain, and an even greater number of synaptic junctions make the contact between them. Thus, at any given moment, trillions of impulses pass from one neuronal cell to another, lighting a perpetual network of activity. This is the inextricable, prodigious infrastructure on which our perceptions, thoughts and emotions are built. Scientists setting up their goal in defining the neurobiological crossroads that lead to subjective states of mind, memory recollections, reasoning and learning are therefore faced with a Herculean task.

Certainly, it is possible to classify various mechanisms of behaviour and analyse the influence played by the environment and inherent genetic factors in these processes. Human cognitive studies, as part of a conglomerate of disciplines composing modern neural science, have succeeded in supplementing important information related to internal representations and the dynamics of mental processes. Nevertheless, despite the existence of an impressive amount of scientific advancements, we are still overwhelmed by the multiplicity of neural mechanisms and quite incapable of establishing a specific correlation between them and the infinite variety of human actions and feelings.

Pertinent to this book is a discussion on brain activities in health, as opposed to disease states, and on the existence of mental capabilities able to enhance healing processes. This cannot be achieved unless we tackle some of the most controversial and intriguing issues confronting today's scientific community: the nature of mind. The great difficulty in suggesting a definition arises not only from the necessity of differentiating between physical and non-physical phenomena, but also from the inability to deal with them as separate entities. How can the mechanics of mental processes be understood, if we do not see clearly into how the brain 'thinks' and 'comprehends', how the image of the 'self' is created, and the role played by consciousness in the appreciation of this image?

Since the earliest days of antiquity, philosophers have made a distinction between animal behaviour, in which natural instincts are prevalent, and human conduct, seen as a result of Man's ability to reason. In modern times, these views have undergone several changes, oscillating, among others, between Freud's definitions of sexual instinct (the need to live), the innate combativeness (the need to die), and behaviourist concepts, unable to conceive the existence of pure instinct without some component of learning or environmental influence.

A complex situation has been identified in which a 'fixed programme' (i.e. the presence of repetitive, stereotypical actions, characteristic of a certain species) coexists with a long list of patterns having their origin in the internal and external environment, and being instrumental in the creation of the final behaviour prototype. Hereditary factors have therefore been studied in order to see how they might influence certain human-conduct traits. A great deal of human performances have been found to be universal, including the presence of what modern psychologists named 'drives' (for example, hunger, thirst, sex and curiosity), and a wide variety of emotional expressions, common to people of different cultures and environments, such as facial expressions of frowning, anger, crying and so on.

To add to the matter's intricacy, the anatomical model of

brain function has identified different specialisations for the right and the left parts of the brain, with most language processing and logical, linear thinking connected to the left hemisphere, and non-verbal, image-related, creative statuses to the right one. Anatomically, communication between the two brain halves is maintained by a connecting structure named the corpus callosum, as well as by nervous fibres forming the anterior and posterior commissures.

With cortical areas in the right hemisphere controlling motor and sensory activities on the left side of the body and vice versa, a normal individual uses both hemispheres. The role of one or another, however, may become predominant, according to specific requirements. For example, the right hemisphere, considered to play an important role in the processing of emotions, can be activated in stress situations, as well as whenever the elaboration of a judgement is necessary.

Moreover, people involved in logical, verbal professions, such as engineers or lawyers, seem to use more often their left-brain capabilities than painters or sculptors, who, on the contrary, need to tap into the imaginative pool of the right brain in order to replenish their creative resources. Recent times have seen a great deal of emphasis placed on right-brain attitudes, meaning the search for a better connection with innate desires and hopes, while 'tuning' to the needs of the self and deriving great practical benefits from it. Still, there is no doubt that the most 'complete' human beings are the ones capable of drawing on both hemispheres' attributes, combining cool, logical reflection with inspired, intuitive actions.

And yet, the above categorisation is not capable of offering us the leverage necessary to understand how mental phenomena occur, and fit in the notion of how to 'mind' with the rest of our known reality. The most faithful approach is probably the one that accepts the existence of several minds, i.e. a diver-

Healing Connections

sity of mental actions based on countless neuronal mechanisms and brain connections, and resulting in as many recognisable memories, thoughts, feelings and decisions. The philosopher Daniel Dennett speaks of 'kinds of minds', when underlining the essence of human consciousness compared with the animal kingdom, as well as the connection of our cognitive tasks with the surrounding environment.

Mental states are different from anything else that we know and are able to appreciate. Essentially, we are dealing with a puzzling maze of phenomena, part of which are conscious and therefore perpetually central to our existence as human beings. On the other hand, the presence of a substantial unconscious component to mental processes only supports the hypothesis that the human mind cannot be explained in physical terms and has most probably a non-physical essence. Thus, not surprisingly, notions such as 'life force', 'vital spark' or 'God-given gift' have been used when referring to human mental characteristics.

In Albert Camus's idea that an intellectual is someone whose mind watches itself (*Notebooks, 1935–42*), our mind is indeed watching itself while it records much of the ongoing thoughts, reasoning processes and emotions. This tip of an iceberg, our consciousness, is defined dryly in dictionaries as 'having the knowledge, the feeling of something', or 'being aware'. The need for an adequate understanding of this intriguing process has resulted in multiple attempts to elucidate its inner mechanics, without being able to propose a unique and fitting model. The subtitle to one of the mathematician Roger Penrose's[*] works hints of the magnitude of the task: 'A search for the missing science of consciousness'.

One of the most tempting and exhilarating possibilities is to

---

[*]Bibliography, p. 121 – Penrose, R.

look at consciousness with a scientific eye, to adapt and apply to mental events the vast knowledge accumulated in the areas of mathematics and physics; to compare the workings of the mind with those of computational systems. Penrose's conclusion is roughly that consciousness, in its particular manifestation in the human quality of 'understanding', is doing something that mere computation cannot. The fact that some aspects of conscious thinking cannot be even simulated by computation, as well as computers being unable to evoke any conscious actions or emotions, conveys the idea that 'the mind must indeed be something that cannot be described in any kind of computational terms'. In his search for a physical connection necessary to explain the non-computability of our conscious mind, Penrose recognises our current inability to propose an adequate scientific concept able to decode the mind's powerfully encrypted messages.

Predictably enough, the study of the subconscious mind becomes a *sine qua non* requirement for an investigation into the workings of the mind. The amalgam of our conscious perceptions, including pains and joys, recent and old memories, likes and dislikes, fears and hopes, has a significant unconscious constituent that takes the most active part in our actions and decision making. Similar to Jean Cocteau's definition of style ('Style is a simple way of saying complicated things', *The Difficulty of Being*), the unconscious has the ability to 'fool' us, i.e. to shelter behind several decodable signals, an extraordinary world of intermingled information, which seems often to escape our introspective awareness.

Considering how well secluded the above domain is, we are at a stage when the 'off-limits to inquiry' suggested by Daniel Dennett may indeed apply to animal mental processes. Here, a great number of 'unconscious' or 'automatic' behaviour patterns have been discovered, and it seems that at the moment we are quite far from being able to appreciate if, for example, there are any 'thoughts' attached to a goldfish's gaze directed from the glass bowl to the child that feeds him. Nevertheless, in the case of human mental activity, some strong allies are there to facilitate the exploratory work. The signature clef represented by the language ability, and the mind's influence on human physiology, are certainly among the most relevant.

Presented for the first time by Darwin as an 'art' with an instinctive component, the language capability is an all-important tool that exerts a tremendous influence on an individual's development, as well as on his or her relationship with others and the surrounding environment. This unique human ability to convey clear messages in particular grammatical forms has been demonstrated to be vitally linked to the existence of sophisticated conscious processes.

The Viennese philosopher Ludwig Wittgenstein, who died in 1951, enjoyed a substantial following based on his studies of the relationship between verbal statements and realities. 'The world is all that is the case,' he declared, focusing on the importance of language in the separation between 'known' and 'unknown' matters. Wittgenstein considered that words construct our sense of reality and, therefore, the world we perceive is only the result of our verbally expressed opinions. We say what we know, we cannot say what we do not know, was the philosopher's main belief. This factual approach, of course, left place for numerous submerged, unfathomable realities without a linguistic coverage but still part of human existence.

Regarding words as representatives of human existence, and appreciating the manner in which they are used, i.e. syntax and context, does not seem to suffice for a comprehensive understanding of the language mechanism. As suggested by the French philosopher Henri-Louis Bergson (1859–1941), viewing consciousness as the working of an *élan vital* (a powerful life force) implies the use of language as a very important connecting instrument between the 'physical body and the non-physical mind'. In many ways, the notion of language could be attached to other parameters, considered by Bergson to represent the essence of reality, and including time, change and development.

More recently, Noam Chomsky's revolutionary linguistic investigations have brought forward the concept of humans being born pre-programmed to use grammatical language. This may explain the speed with which young children learn to speak, and implies the fact that they must have in place neural structures already configured to process certain types of information. As much as Chomsky's work, and that of other contemporary investigators, has explained part of the evolutionary mysteries of the human brain, we are still left with some of the main queries raised already in the seventeenth century by René Descartes, the illustrious French philosopher and mathematician who initiated much of the modern study of the mind and consciousness.

Based on a dualism that the material human body and the insubstantial mind are two different things, Descartes wondered how it was possible that thoughts arose from physical matter. If physical substance is completely separated from thought, where then is the mind located? If it is not material, in what way does it exist? And how does it interact with the human body and the surrounding world? These, and other similarly important questions, were grouped under the name 'the mind–body problem', an enigma that continues to be of paramount contemporary interest, even though the current scientific tendency has clearly distanced itself from Descartes's logical and religious grounds.

Due to the unreliable nature of our sensual input, subjective experience is not satisfactory, and human accepted knowledge is doubtful, further noticed Descartes. Consequently, he proposed a way of improving the collective comprehension, by confirming human existence as proper to a thinking creature. *Cogito ergo sum*, he said, I think, therefore I am. To the belief that the world's substance may be a mirage, a misrepresentation brought forward by a possibly faulty human logic, Descartes opposed the idea of thinking as the foundation of all truth. Irrelevant to how we envisage reality, he remarked, the fact that we think about the issue makes its presence tangible and true.

The following centuries, however, have seen a clear weakening in Descartes's approach, as scientific works have replaced the pursuit of an absolute truth with partial and temporary verities, subject to experimental change. Such analytical trials have been proven useful especially in the shadowy domain of the human unconscious, where a great deal of verification is needed.

As suggested by Descartes, the power of thought enables us to elaborate on symbolic entities, connected both to our personal identity and to the infinite variety of objects surrounding us. In other words, we do have the possibility of clearly separating the self-conscious 'I' from the formative social reality revealed by our minds. Most human life circumstances firmly perpetuate this division, which results in an intricate and fluctuating need to break such dualism, whenever an adjustment, a better comprehension or a liberation from stereotypes is required.

With its characteristic emphasis on the concrete, our existence becomes therefore interspersed with numerous more or less successful attempts to overcome the difficulties created by the demands for survival, social integration and profitable actions. Deep-rooted emotions play an important part in the final shaping of those performances, a fact that has constantly attracted the attention of researchers of the mind.

Sigmund Freud spoke about the latent, potential ability to become knowledgeable about events and objects that we are currently unaware of. 'The conscious mind may be compared to a fountain playing in the sun and falling back into the great subterranean pool of unconscious from which it rises,' said Freud in *Die Traumdeutung* (*The Interpretation of Dreams*). His ground-breaking assumption that in the subconscious mind an immense store of information is there for us to delve into, if only we could find the appropriate means of probing it, has revolutionised the general view of how the mind works. As a novel concept, it influenced contemporary brain science to such a degree that consciousness and the unconscious today form in our eyes inseparable aspects of mental phenomena.

Based on his studies on hysteria, and while using dream analysis as a clinical technique, the acclaimed psychologist also introduced the notions of 'super-ego' (the idealist view of self, including moral duties and faith), 'ego' (the part of the mind that develops from our sensorial perceptions and our interaction with the external world) and the 'id' (the shadowy, impulsive core of interior experiences).

As chief constituents of an individual's mental setup, these factors have a decisive power in the creation of the unconscious, based on the permanent opposition between the ego's tendency to react to the demands of the practical world ('the reality principle'), and the id's willingness to follow only instinctual desires ('the pleasure principle'). While suggesting that the information released from the innermost recesses of our mind is less significant than that which is held back, Freud recognised mental activities as being at the heart of a prodigious struggle between inner and outer influences.

This idea of a continuous clash between, on one side, the

instinctive need to live, the fear of dying or the sexual urges, and, on the other, the circumstances of social realities, became widely accepted and was to be repeated, refined and also distorted, many times after its introduction. The famous child psychoanalyst Melanie Klein, for example, strongly influenced by Sigmund Freud, took further the principle of inner, emotion-laden influences and concluded that the external world plays only a secondary role in the psychological makeup of a child.

Such a principle of a crucial internal origin of the active psychic life of an individual is easily transferable to a biophysical level, where a great number of imbalances were demonstrated to be the result of hidden conflicts and to arrive at conscious expression in the form of an abnormal behaviour pattern or disguised under disease symptoms. The autonomic nervous system is extremely sensitive to the presence of chronic stress or emergency stress situations, during which it becomes active and cooperates with various glands in the human organism, especially the adrenals.

The release of chemical products, including adrenaline, noradrenalin and various steroids, creates a chain reaction in which, among others, the heart rate and the blood sugar are increased, blood clots move faster, the blood pressure augments and there is white-cell hyperactivity. All these occurrences, when taking place for short periods of time, have no nocive effects and constitute healthy defensive body mechanisms. However, if the stress situation continues, practically any system in the body, the immune, the circulatory or the digestive, will suffer from its inability to cope with the destructive changes.

Clinical experience has demonstrated that countless diseases, ranging from hypertension to diabetes, and including cancers, heart attacks and strokes, have their roots in an impaired mind–body connection, i.e. in the activation of brain mechanisms capable of exerting a detrimental influence on the body's well-being. The complex neuronal and chemical pathways at the base of these phenomena have not yet been completely elucidated. What is clearly known, however, is the fact that pharmacological therapy in the form of an ever-increasing line of drugs does not seem to be of great benefit in these illnesses.

Attempting to find a solution to the problem is more complicated than it seems. Historical successes achieved by modern medical science, cannot be overlooked and, despite the recent proliferation of alternative therapeutic approaches, there is no realistic opportunity for their success without a solid factual and experimentally verified backing. Most importantly, the necessity has arisen for the core issue of the mind–body relationship to be clarified in a manner that will satisfy criteria of both age-long healing traditions in various cultures around the globe and conventional Western-type medical criteria.

Finding a balance between the two comprises a radical revision of fundamental approaches to biological processes, the workings of the mind and life in general. Alfred Whitehead, the co-author with Bertrand Russell of *Principia Mathematica*, an important work on the logical foundations of mathematics, has advised us to look at the world, on physical, biological and psychological levels, as a process of continuous activity and regeneration. Therefore, to immobilise the process and analyse separated parts of it will offer only a very restricted view.

Taking this into consideration, it is possible to understand why the revival of the concept of a mind–body mechanism having a physiological influence stirs so much argument. The modern medical environment, based on over-specialisation, with all its evident benefits of high skill and performance, seems to have gradually alienated the modern practitioner and researcher from the comprehensive inquiring view.

It is as if the extensive accumulated knowledge on the brain's anatomical structure holds back the exploratory work, since it predisposes researchers to preconceived ideas about localisation of processes. The portrayal of the human brain as an organic computer programmed over millions of years belongs to the same attitude of envisaging the mind as a compendium of neural activity specialising in performing specific tasks.

Fiercely attacked by those who refuse to see the human spirit reduced to a sequence of nervous impulses, this viewpoint can be found clearly with Freud, who subscribed entirely to the significance of probing the thought content of an individual. For him, our senses are the main source of information from the physical reality. Moreover, this information has to be placed in a rational framework in order to be credited with any meaning.

After him, the subject has been widely and actively pursued, with some authors regarding mental properties as physical attributes of the brain, and others, while still considering them as real phenomena, believing that they are completely distinct from material functions. The angles of approach are also diverse, with conclusions extrapolated either from clinical studies or from philosophical musings over the issue.

In recent years, a great deal of hope has been placed on an imaging technique named positron emission tomography (PET), which enables doctors to follow metabolic processes in the brain. This is achieved by recording the progress of a radioactive chemical injected or inhaled by the patient. Different levels of activity in specific brain areas have been correlated with medical conditions, such as Parkinson's disease, schizophrenia or Alzheimer's disorder. The same method is currently employed to study memory patterns and grammatical language processing, as well as musical imagery and perception.

In relation with brain activity, it is interesting to mention that in the search for relaxation responses able to induce a healing, restorative status, mental sound processing may be of undeniable importance. Modern researchers are currently exploring the place of auditory stimuli such as chants, drum beating or the repetition of specific words (mantra) in the preparation for meditative states and the creation of altered states of consciousness, well known, as we will see further on, in shamanic and Eastern healing traditions. Studies performed by MP Rogers *et al.* in 1979, and appearing in the journal *Psychosomatic Medicine*, as well as findings by other authors, such as MP Anderson or H Benson have shown clear physiological benefits occurring during such events, including a reduction in the heart rate and blood pressure, lessened muscular tension and an increase in the alpha and theta activity on the EEG (recorded electrical activity of the brain). Theta brain waves, especially, have been demonstrated to be related to states of increased creativity and vivid imagination.

Eminent researchers, including A Neher, J Khalfa, S Arom and others, have studied the effects of sound on the human brain in various ways, ranging from the investigation of the structural components of music perception, to works exploring the musical traditions of African or South-American societies, and clinical observations on relaxation responses. It seems that by repeated, monotonous stimulation of the auditory pathways, a typical mental state or a change in cognitive awareness is produced, which heightens the pain threshold, promotes restfulness and concentration, and most probably assists in bypassing the logical, verbal part of our consciousness towards the veiled intuitive resources.

In addition, sound has been shown to act as a device that greatly facilitates visualisation, with all its implications of positive imagery used as a healing tool. Siding with John Keats, who said in a letter to Benjamin Bailey, 'I am certain of nothing but the holiness of the heart's affections and the truth of imagination' (*Letter to Benjamin Bailey, 1817*), it has been pointed out that mental images, able to displace themselves from the surrounding environment and recreate wishes, can mediate between conscious desires and the physical status. A special ritual of self-control and reinforcement can thus be created in support of an individual's need to augment his or her body's natural healing abilities.

The study of this issue can certainly shed light on the states of consciousness favouring medical cures, as well as support the continuous search for the recondite mystery of the soul, notoriously seen with Tibetan monks or Jewish mystics. The subject is of great scientific interest as well, with some eminent researchers devoting their investigations to this area, including the co-discoverer of the structure of DNA and Nobel Prize winner, Francis Crick. Some of his views, as expressed in the book *The Astonishing Hypothesis*, as well as in some of the correspondence which I had the great privilege of exchanging with him, will be discussed in the next two chapters. They deal with Man's age-long and harrowing search for his veritable nature, as a component of an infinite life-chain in a highly mysterious universe.

Chapter 2

An Infinite Sphere

Nature, to be commanded, must be obeyed.
Francis Bacon, *Novum Organum*

The insatiable urge to explore the surrounding habitat and to question its origin relentlessly is as old as humanity. In view of the innumerable attempts to formulate an effective explanation both for our existence on this planet and the existence of the universe in general, it is appropriate to quote the British essayist William Hazlitt, who considered that 'the most fluent talkers or most plausible reasoners are not always the justest thinkers.' (*Sketches and Essays "On Prejudice"*)

Powerful biological concepts have been invoked to justify and explain the overwhelming variety of organic and inorganic material on earth. The evolutionary key appeared for a time sufficiently sophisticated to fit into a great number of locks and open hitherto tightly closed doors of knowledge. Up to the present day, many believe in a gradual unfolding of natural history, including the shaping of the universe from the initial Big Bang to its present state, including the development of increasingly sophisticated life forms on earth.

Calculated to have occurred some three and a half billion years ago, the prehistoric emergence of living organisms initiated a relentless perfecting process. It spanned simple, ocean-located, bacteria-like cells, through to algae and protozoans, and to complex multicellular organisms such as fish, insects, plants, reptiles, birds and mammals. The origins of the human species, however, remain clouded in uncertainty and continue to represent a vivid subject of debate.

Skeletons of the earliest known human ancestors have been found in the Ethiopian and Kenyan deserts. Named *Australopithecus ramidus* and *Australopithecus afarensis*, these creatures were characterised by upright walking and have been dated as living some four million years ago. They are most probably the ancestors of *Homo habilis*, the user of stones as first utensils, and of *Homo erectus*, who discovered the use of fire and, less than two million years ago, eventually moved out of Africa.

Modern humans, named *Homo sapiens*, together with the large-brained and heavily built Neanderthals, are believed to have descended from *Homo erectus*. The Neanderthals populated the European continent and the Middle East during the Ice Age, after which they slowly disappeared some forty thousand years ago, leaving behind *Homo sapiens* as the sole modern representative of the hominid species.

Numerous details of this lengthy procession of events, however, are still uncertain. Recent molecular studies, including DNA analysis in human populations, support a theory according to which a common African ancestor, living some two hundred thousand years ago, is at the origin of modern humans, who spread throughout the world from Africa. On the other hand, there are scientists who believe that a complex selection process took place, not only in Africa, but in multiple centres around the world, resulting in the development of advanced forms of *Homo sapiens* everywhere on the planet.

Even if an agreement exists among scientists on the idea that human populations separated some fifty to one hundred thousand years ago into today's recognised groups (Asian, European, Australasian, etc.), no understanding exists on how from these Neolithic precursors an extraordinary cultural explosion took place around 6,000 BC, resulting in the rise of numerous highly civilised societies around the globe, such as the Mesopotamian, the Chinese, the Olmec and many others.

No satisfactory explanation has been provided as yet for the lack of evidence of 'intermediary' developmental stages of these ancient communities, logically necessary to occur, before evolved writing and mathematical abilities, engineering skills and highly sophisticated astronomical and medical knowledge would emerge. This missing connection points to the continuous mystery surrounding the beginning of human life on earth but is not a dilemma for creationists, however, who believe in the presence of a superior, universal and immortal power, responsible for all acts of creation, including that of earth's first inhabitants.

It is not surprising that the uncertainty related to his veritable provenance created in Man an inner turmoil, normally and permanently reflected in his social interactions, as well as in his cultural and artistic expressions. This uncertainty continued to underline the value of human intellect, being the only means of probing the intricacies of life and, ultimately, serving as the most powerful connector to the enigmas of nature.

Early in a sinuous and revelatory process, people faced the realisation that while living on this planet, animals, plants and the unpredictable climatic whims all had to be taken into account as meaningful partners. An imperative need for a successful integration followed, which required constant vigilance, observation, comparison and an appropriate exploitation of beneficial circumstances.

With time, the terrestrial sphere became less and less foreign to Man, who, during his agitated and substantial history, encountered innumerable opportunities to demonstrate a frequent superiority, but also occasional highly disappointing limitations vis-à-vis other environmental competitors. Soon enough, an awareness of inescapable mortality began to haunt humans; an uneasy feeling of being merely short-lived visitors amidst the beautiful, rich and perpetually changing decorum of nature. This perception fuelled a continuous search for a world beyond their own, and resulted in a relentless tendency to cling on to matters of infinity.

The extraordinary scientific discoveries of recent times have succeeded in clarifying many long-standing queries. Einstein's genius brought forward the theory of relativity, in the process disrupting many preconceived notions concerning the workings of the universe. By stating that mass and motion have a relative, rather than absolute, characteristic, and that matter, time and space are interdependent, Einstein's ideas very much opened the way for a long line of revelations of great theoretical and practical value.

As a result, a new and continuously changing view of reality has emerged, in which an enormous amount of perplexing paradoxes are still awaiting resolution. They include the ability to correlate classical Newtonian physics with the astonishing conclusions of quantum mechanics, or to combine the latter with the presence of relativity.

An example of the magnitude, importance and considerably confusing character of the quest is the superstring theory, developed in 1980. It describes the interplay between elementary particles and the nuclear and gravity forces. In this concept, primary objects in the universe are viewed as being exceedingly small and stringlike, rather than, as previously thought, pointlike.

The simply mind-boggling conclusion of this theory is that the existence of such objects implies the prevalence of a ten-dimension universe. For reasons not yet understood, only three space dimensions and one dimension of time are perceivable at the moment. To add to the complexity of the issue, there has been academic discussion about the possible presence of multiple universes; ones in which photons (light particles), whose existence may be dependent on an observer watching them, can be in two places at once, travel faster than light and move backwards in time.

It is not surprising, therefore, that in view of the astounding recent disclosures, a vivid and refuelled recognition developed of the limited human capacity to grasp a larger-than-life reality. Recent manned travel to outer space, while enlarging our visibility of neighbouring stars and planets, seems only to add more weight to a sense of great humility in the face of (in the words of Stephen Hawking in *A Brief History of Time*), 'an endless and ever-expanding universe'.

It is therefore highly intriguing to muse on Plato's remark in *Theaetetus* that 'Man is the measure for all things'. One way to understand this is as a fundamental concept stating that the human microcosm is comparable, or even identical with, the unlimited and magnificent macrocosm. This idea can be found reverberating in numerous ancient traditions such as the Jewish Kabbalah ('as above so below'), or the Chinese and Indian philosophical doctrines. While strongly supporting the belief in a spiritual dimension to human existence, all these teachings include a coherent and definite position towards a unified perspective, i.e. the recognition of a highly interdependent and harmonious life phenomenon.

Healing Connections

This principle grows to great significance when the Cartesian split between mind and matter is taken into consideration. As mentioned in the previous chapter, historically, numerous scientific and philosophical attempts have been made to unravel the confusing issue of the relationship between the two categories. Modern thinking, as we have seen, has the tendency to turn more and more towards the acceptance of a single cognitive network as the base of human consciousness, and therefore away from Descartes's original ideas.

Unable to fully comprehend the workings of his own mind, Man arrived at the conclusion that it may be easier, while free from the strait-jacket of subjectivity, to first decipher the rules governing the surrounding world. Hence, daring and ground-breaking scientific discoveries occurring along the passing centuries brought humanity to a level of understanding that is both evolved and multi-focused. Advanced intellectual concepts currently encompass all that is intimately connected to one's existence: time, space, personal identity, as well as relationships with other human beings and nature itself.

A new conceptual standpoint has developed in which reality is perceived as a network of interrelated events, involving both the finite human body and the gigantic, everlasting universe. This appears to be in strong contradistinction with the traditional train of thought promoted by pioneering anatomists and physiologists, who saw the human organism as a compendium of independently working systems, as well as by astronomers, mathematicians and physicists, who embraced a similar, 'mechanical' and dissociated view of the cosmos.

Nowadays, it has become common to discuss the presence of interlacing ecosystems, of space and time entwined into a

The Human Hologram

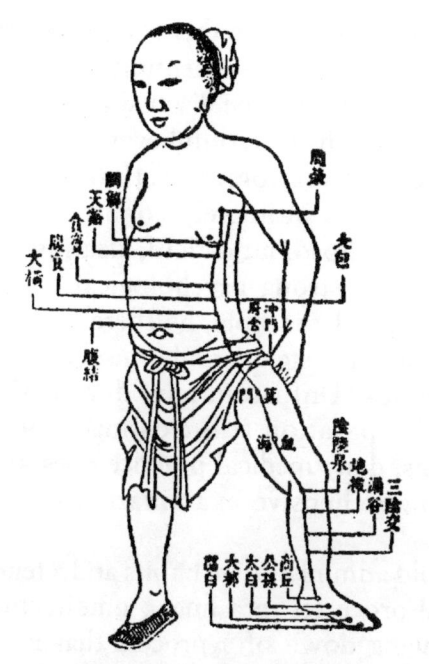

Chinese acupuncture points

single entity, and of a phenomenal matrix of life, possibly extending well beyond our own world. In this perspective, it is easy to understand the necessity of reviewing some of medicine's basic principles relating to the treatment of both organic and psychological ailments. Mainly, healing processes should be understood as complex occurrences involving concomitant mental, emotional and biological activities.

The body's defence mechanisms, the capabilities of tissue repair and regeneration, as well as the generalised control over a multitude of functions are provided by a variety of systems working in unison. A special place among them is occupied by the immune network, which has been shown to be very sensitive to minimal changes in the organism's status quo, and capable of reacting to them in unexpected and intricate ways. The subject will be mentioned again in the third part of the book, when I will be discussing ways of improving the body's capacity to fight harmful events.

Virtually every physiological activity, far from being an isolated process, is intimately connected to the rest of the body. The psychosomatic field, dealing with organic diseases that have a strong psychological component, represents such a typical example, as there is an involvement of several functional systems, and consequently, of various clinical disciplines. Unfortunately, due to the persistent and quite rigid separation still existing between different medical domains, daily medical practice does not adequately allow for a comprehensive examination of an individual patient.

Entrenched old administrative habits and a tendency to perceive biological processes in a linear, unidirectional manner, add to the slowing down of a process that is, nevertheless, inexorably advancing towards the unification of medical judgement and a broader approach to diagnosis and therapy. Developed many centuries ago by the majority of ancient human societies, the idea of a harmonious and balanced approach to the disease process, of *primo non nocere* (firstly do not harm) and, in general, of an earthly and human destiny closely mirroring the cosmological unfolding, is being rediscovered by our contemporaries.

Thoughts and words, our ancestors considered, are imbued with creative and healing powers. They should be used carefully and only in an altruistic and compassionate context. Moreover, while chaos and disorder are the main propagators of illness and human misery, attunement to the regulatory vibrations of nature carries a perpetual blessing for health and wholeness.

In the teachings of reputable scientists the indispensable connection with nature can be found as a repetitive leitmotiv. Hippocrates, the Greek physician living around 400 BC, and considered to be the father of medicine, advised in *Precepts* that 'we must turn to nature itself, to the observations of the body in health and disease in order to learn the truth'; Paracelsus, the fifteenth-century Swiss doctor and alchemist, recognised in *Seven Defences* that 'the art of healing comes from nature not from the physician, therefore the physician must start from nature with an open mind'; and, in our era, Werner Heisenberg (1901–76), the German physicist who developed the revolutionary quantum theory, stated 'natural science does not simply describe and explain nature, it is part of the interplay between nature and ourselves.' (*Physics and Philosophy*)

The increased communication ability in the extended family of Man has brought with it the clear advantage of observation and learning, with an often unsuspected and bewildering recognition of similarities. Aspirations, fears, joys and pains seem to have a universal, basic human content that is both unifying and secluding. Unifying, as the exhibition of characteristic qualities and limitations has brought humanity towards an increased identity awareness. People see themselves as possessors of a similar makeup, which represents their only ammunition against adverse circumstances coming from outside their known world. Secluding, as Man is required to assess his position continuously in relation to surrounding nature and, while inquisitively gazing into the infinite mirror of a starry sky, he seems to perceive an image that is not his own. Thus the perennial questions of 'who am I?' and 'what is the purpose of my existence on this planet?' remain nowadays as meaningful as ever.

Moreover, humanity advances towards an appreciation of

Healing Connections

self-reliance, taking charge of its own destiny and the capability to actively participate at the shaping of the future. Being able to conquer illness, disability and ageing represents an integral part of this tremendously complicated and arduous process. In its unfolding, learning the immutable laws of nature is an essential step towards the formation of a valuable and rewarding partnership.

In the words of Walt Whitman:

> The earth does not argue,
> Is not pathetic, has no arrangements,
> Does not scream, haste, persuade, threaten, promise,
> Makes no discriminations, has no conceivable failures,
> Closes nothing, refuses nothing, shuts none out.

Together with knowledge, mankind can extract extraordinary measures of balance, humility and strength. These invaluable qualities have the potential to serve as a reliable and necessary powerhouse designed to propel humanity towards a better future.

Chapter 3

Acting As Man: the Machine Barrier

The Universe begins to look more like a great thought than like a great machine.

James Jeans, *The Mysterious Universe*

René Descartes, the seventeenth-century French philosopher and mathematician, remarked that the most intelligent animal belongs to a different category than the least intelligent human being. Such a position takes us immediately to the search for a better comprehension of the word 'intelligence'. The conventional biological and physical nature of Man places him, as we have seen, in the top rank of a continuous chain of development. Physical characteristics would certainly not be sufficient for the attainment of this prestigious standing, as numerous animals can pride themselves on being larger, stronger, faster and possessing capabilities of which human beings are totally deprived, for example, flying or breathing under water.

What is recognised under the term 'human superiority' usually reflects the admission that Man is endowed with specific mental and psychological traits that allow him to perceive and judge reality, grasp abstract notions, seek explanations and, all along these processes, substantially change his environment. We have already explored the demonstrated distinctions between Man and members of the animal kingdom. The recent technological revolution has, however, added a new dimension to the pursuit for a clarification and definition of what is termed as 'intelligent behaviour': the introduction of artificial intelligence (AI).

There are few who have better summarised the concept of AI than Marvin Minsky, founder of the Artificial Intelligence Laboratory at the Massachusetts Institute of Technology (MIT): 'Artificial Intelligence is the science of making machines do things that would require intelligence if done by men.'

After the first digital computers became operational in the 1940s, several subsequent generations of these highly performing machines have resulted in the well-known, general-purpose computer and a level of sophistication that allows the performance of innumerable intellectual tasks traditionally considered as being unique to humans. Thus electronic brains can store facts in the form of numbers or characters, then retrieve, arrange, rearrange, classify and analyse this information. They can perform exceedingly complex calculations and be theoretically programmed to solve any problem for which a solution can be found based on the same given data.

Alan Turing, the English mathematician and logician, described in 1936 a 'universal computing machine' that could become a very powerful aid to scientific, technological and social advancement. He was also the founding father of the philosophy of artificial intelligence. Subjecting the question:

Can machines think? to a heated philosophical debate, Turing opened an era where technological advancements would be continuously scrutinised for their ability to compare with humans. Even more importantly, the question would be raised on how the study of computers could tell us more about our own nature.

Nowadays a fully developed branch of science, artificial intelligence deals with the creation of computer programs that can perform actions comparable to those of an intelligent human. Successes are numerous, with an almost daily improvement in the achieved aptitudes. Still, there is a great persistent dilemma regarding the ability of human thought to be grasped as a set of formal instructions which, in the case of a computer, is processed as information. The direct reasoning would seem to be that if the human mind could be entirely reduced to such instructions, then it is easy to assume that a 'well-informed' machine could be considered as having a 'mind'. Controversial as it is, the matter is of profound interest not only to theoreticians, but also to those who attempt to identify the practical benefits from an increased use of 'thinking machines'.

From one point of view, it is not possible to reduce thought to a summation of mechanical parameters, just as, on the contrary, it is difficult to explain intricate mental phenomena such as love, hate, pain or joy as being much more than the result of the activity of chemical neurotransmitters and neural impulses in the brain. Current AI research has been advancing well in such domains as mathematical intelligence, language understanding, pattern recognition and knowledge representation. At the same time, wide areas including communication, error appreciation, choice making and cognition seem to remain complex and lie outside the capabilities of computers.

The central question is precisely how human intellectual activity escapes mechanical imprisonment. The implications of brainstorming, organisation of ideas and demonstration of creativity are enhanced by the all-important but hidden therapeutic potential. Modern times have seen the inclusion of computers into all areas of human activities. The prodigious variety of their uses and the ever-increasing complexity of their tasks undoubtedly mirror the evolution in human thought. While constructing computer-activated robots able to replace human labour, as well as facing issues such as whether highly performing machines can rightfully be called 'electronic brains' and whether we are computers, humanity has been given the opportunity to engage on a very important path of advanced self-discovery.

Perhaps the most important notion to ponder is the ability to feel, i.e. to react to certain situations or sensory stimuli, an ability that remains inherent to humans and, in the view of most researchers, will never be attained by a man-made machine. We are all familiar with the emotional effect of the sight of a beautiful sunset, the smell of a rose or the cry of a child. Preserving his natural possession of aesthetic criteria and a whole gamut of sensations, Man can proudly investigate what exactly makes the difference.

Eliza, the artificial-intelligence program created at MIT by Joseph Weizenbaum, can well serve as an example. Named after Eliza Doolittle, the character in Bernard Shaw's play *Pygmalion*, the program was, as in the play's plot, taught by the professor to speak exceedingly well and to reply to inquisitive remarks. To the programmer's great surprise, Eliza soon became a highly sought-after 'psychotherapist', with people finding their 'guiding' sessions with her invaluable, completely ignoring the fact that she was not a real person. In Weizenbaum's own words: 'I had not realised that extremely short exposures to a relatively simple computer program could induce powerful delusional thinking in quite normal people.'

This story is representative of the current tendency of empowering machines with human qualities. As with HAL, the computer featured in *Space Odyssey: 2001*, it is often perceived that other machines could also be switching from automatic, controlled behaviour, to authority and independent decision making. Moreover, a great deal of human welfare is entrusted nowadays to computers. Excluding the possibility of inherent technical failures, considerable doubts still exist concerning the ability of 'thinking machines' to fully comprehend human problems and innermost feelings. As advanced and sophisticated as these computers may seem, it seems that the changes take place mainly in the human psyche, only too eager to accept mechanical control over its affairs.

Can robots save this troubled world? This is a recurrent question that has strong reverberations in the medical field, where computer programs are already utilised in the diagnostic process. By introducing into the computer's memory all data pertinent to the patient's medical history, current complaints, as well as findings of various examinations, a physician expects to receive a detailed and final diagnosis, to be taken seriously into consideration when deciding on the appropriate treatment. Nevertheless, in numerous medical centres objection has been voiced against the regular and uncompromising acceptance of this method, which excludes the dimension added by the doctor's invaluable personal experience and intuition.

In specifically considering human awareness or consciousness, we arrive at the conclusion that something very important and unique separates Man from programmed machines. First of all, there is the perception of the exterior world that is processed by Man's sensory organs through a complex physiological and psychological process. For example, light reflected from the sun stimulates the specialised rod and cone cells in the eye, with a further effect on the cerebral cortex and the resulting visual sensation.

Additionally, the sun's light may trigger a cascade of contingent feelings such as well-being, warmth, relaxation or, on the contrary, a need for increased activity. While a computer can also elicit a range of items associated with a specific object, there is always a limit to the number of components entered by the programmer from the beginning. In contrast, with a human being, one can often arouse an unexpected reaction. For instance, the perception of light can mean that the night is over and a new working day is about to begin, thus frequently inducing a rather unpleasant sensation.

This example gives occasion for an additional argument, that of the human disposition, highly influencing the perception of reality.

> To see the World in a grain of sand,
> And a Heaven in a wild flower,
> Hold Infinity in the palm of your hand,
> And Eternity in an hour...

William Blake's words, from 'Auguries of Innocence', reflect strongly the nature of the human mind, able to transpose into material existence its own images, its original mind-made objects. From here the path towards self-knowledge is consistently made difficult by the infinite possibilities, the complex, astonishing, often quite unbelievable concoctions of an individual mind. This point is best illustrated later in the book, when I will attempt to search for the most appropriate mind-control techniques in what is mostly an overwhelming variety of individual mental cores.

To a large extent, contemporary views on the nature of the human mind and its reproduction by electronic devices originate in the theories of such illustrious thinkers as Plato, Aristotle and Descartes, who supported the concept of a thinking entity separated from the physical body. Descartes attempted to suggest the pineal gland, a centrally located brain structure, as a possible site, but did not have much scientific confirmation at the time. Nevertheless, as we have previously seen, his famous *cogito ergo sum* (I think therefore I am) summarises in the most simple, elegant and convincing manner the complete dependency of human consciousness on its ability to grasp reality.

Unfortunately, even modern science has not yet been able to provide the arguments necessary for a conclusive definition. As we have seen, in an era of vertiginous technical advancements, forced into searching for a reply as to human mental capabilities, brain activity has been likened to computational systems. In lieu of something more substantial, researchers have compromised on concentrating their studies on human intellectual competence. They have described, much in the Platonic tradition, the realms capable of being objectively investigated by Man.

They include the world of nature or the physical world, which contains all that surrounds us, from a table to a butterfly or a distant star. Then, the mathematical world, which has its origin in the ancient belief expressed by Pythagoras, the Greek mathematician living around 500 BC, that the structure of the world, as well as the way to all truth and understanding, is hidden in the knowledge of numbers. Clearly described later by Plato, the mathematical sphere has a strong connection with the visible, tangible world. Nevertheless, the only way a human being is able to have a glimpse of all the worlds, of the totality of existence, is by activating the mysterious mental world, the clue to his personal essence.

As heavily metaphysical and impenetrable as it seems, a contemplation of Man's mental abilities, of his genuine mental powers, can only be beneficial for a harmonious and appropriate development of humanity, despite environmental changes and technical evolution. Both the subtle physical ingredients of our brain being scrutinised by neuroscience, and psychologists and psychiatrists attempting to clarify the patterns of human behaviour, should provide enough evidence to come to terms with mathematics and the body of knowledge resulting from technical experimentation and the manufacturing of robots.

We will then be able to better understand why there are various levels of conscious comprehension and sensitivity, with some of us having an increased ability to 'see' and reproduce beauty, to create unique objects or to fathom original ideas. Moreover, we can learn how to use the unmistakable powers of thought existing in each of us to improve our condition, fulfil our aspirations and develop a sense of wonder and appreciation in the face of the masterful complexity of nature.

Ultimately, much of the essence of the mind remains a mystery, and the comparison with computers only adds to its magnitude. However, as Einstein mentioned in *The World as I See It*, published in 1931: 'The most beautiful experience we can have is the mysterious. It is the fundamental emotion that stands at the cradle of true art and true science.' Searching to gain the upper hand in the competition with our own intellectual faculties is a mission that fully supports this view.

Chapter 4

Soul Searching

> We cannot kindle when we will
> The fire that in the heart resides
> The spirit bloweth and is still,
> In mystery our soul abides.
>
> Matthew Arnold, *Morality*

Around the year 350 BC, the greatest of the Greek orators, Demosthenes, is said to have walked around with a lit candle searching for truth – the eternal truth, that is, the complete and unmovable truth, capable of offering humanity, once and for ever, a glimpse into the mysterious designs of the world. Today, a great many years later, and following numerous scientific revelations, the elusive verity so arduously pursued seems to have vanished even further into the limitless ocean of knowledge.

As seen in the previous chapters, the intricate and almost painfully difficult riddle to solve, that of our consciousness, has continued to preoccupy philosophers and psychologists, as well as members of the exact sciences group. None of the tentative approaches proposed until now seems to have completely fenced in a stable and comprehensive definition. Most of the time, various individual brain functions and psychological characteristics have been studied, in the hope that these secondary doors, when opened, would lead towards a clear and straightforward path into the interminable and shady labyrinth of the spiritual world.

One by one, and with only partial success, topics such as language and visual capabilities, or personal and social behavioural patterns, have been intensely analysed for their likelihood in providing a clue to the unfathomable properties of the human mind and its potential to uncover the mysteries of the universe. However, for the flesh and blood Man, scientific theories represent irrelevant components of daily life. Most of the discussed issues sound incomprehensible and unfamiliar to people accustomed only to the input assembled from their senses. Sounds, images, feelings and innermost yearnings make up human life to such an extent that all information, abstract enough not to be verifiable by sensory perception, automatically becomes classified as impersonal and suspicious.

The logical conclusion, therefore, would be that while attempting to escape the terrifying evidence of one's mortality, as well as searching for support and protection in the preponderant life struggle, Man would not worship things that he cannot see or feel. As everybody knows, this assumption is opposed to reality.

While creating innumerable images of gods to be revered, in the form of statues and other objects of worship, people of all cultures have developed since the dawn of time a belief in the existence of another world, different from that of the senses, and not directly accessible by them. They imagined this world populated by complex, unseen and omnipotent deities, the actions of which have been described in countless myths and legends.

These myths, which involve occasional face-to-face encounters with divine heroes, contain an underlying belief in the presence of an overpowering, invisible and immortal force in charge of human destiny. Thus a great number of mystical beliefs can be described as purely 'religions of the mind', as the only possibility of transcending the given limits of the material world and connecting to the spiritual source is by using one's intellect, i.e. attempting to employ one's mind to understand God's essence and, while doing so, hoping to adapt its standards to human life.

Along the centuries collective rituals have added a strong backing to individual aspirations and, as a result, human qualities such as enhanced perception, wisdom, unselfishness and courage came to be attributed to a very special and highly revered dimension of human existence: that of having a soul. The idea fully supports the perpetual human quest for an integration into the universal wheel of nature, and also offers a welcome opportunity to envisage one's fleeting lifespan as a unique and eternal spark, originating and connected to a divine blaze, the source of all creation.

Researchers of the seventeenth century held deeply religious beliefs. A good example is Isaac Newton who, together with his extraordinary scientific insights, expressed an unfailing certitude in the existence of a supreme, governing force, whose main principles people were only beginning to decipher. While stating that the earth and all heavenly bodies are linked together by a common origin and the same physical laws, Newton promoted a dualistic view, which divided reality into two substances, matter and mind.

Matter and mind were considered by the Dutch philosopher

Baruch Spinoza as the basic modes of expression of an infinite substance called God or Nature. In this way, greatly influenced by Descartes's mathematical approach to the structure of the universe, he supported the idea, soon to be embraced by other thinkers, of a rationalistic pantheism. This doctrine, whose name comes from the Greek *pan* (all), and *theos* (God), regards all reality as divine, and God's presence inherent to all of nature and the entire universe.

At the same time, biological foundations for the existence of the soul were difficult, if not impossible to find. Descartes's idea of the soul being centrally located in the human brain, in the pineal gland, lost ground almost immediately, as it could not be demonstrated in practice. Forms of spiritual quest, however, continued to exist, and combined popular rites and worldwide religious traditions with scientific modes of inquiry, which attempted to provide an edifying testimony for the existence of a spiritual domain underlying the physical world.

The journey beyond the self, so ardently directed by endless generations of humans towards the finding of the ultimate truth, has a very strong and clear psychological provenance, as it offers a unique chance of establishing a point of enduring stability in the universal, bewildering whirl. Thus, at the twilight zone between the physical world and immateriality, humanity has fervently embraced various forms of spiritual attunement to a higher power, considered to govern both nature and man and, consequently, capable of offering comfort in times of adversity.

It is possible, therefore, to comprehend why the founder of existentialism, the Danish philosopher and theologian Søren Kierkegaard, considered that no system of thought is comparable to the unique experience of an individual. People have to overcome their essential concerns, mainly the fear of dying and the feeling of loneliness in an arbitrary universe, but at the same time they are endowed with free will and, as such, are able to affect the course of passing events in their lives. Man's free will, and the manner in which nature reacts to human input, constitute a raging and as yet unresolved divergence of opinions, between scientists who believe in a Newtonian-type model of a perfectly designed and neatly ordered world, and those who, like the eminent physicists Niels Bohr and Werner Heisenberg, are followers of the principle of chaos or indeterminism.

According to the chaos theory, in the invisible and minute world of atoms and subatomic structures, nature's behaviour is capricious, uncertain and greatly influenced by human interference and observation. This path-breaking principle implies that, for example, a photon (the basic unit in which light is emitted) becomes 'real', i.e. comes into existence, only after being observed and measured. Thus one cannot predict the moment-to-moment behaviour of the components of an atomic system and, in general, it is unwarranted to describe a particle's measured parameters as definite and unchangeable.

Inconceivable as it may seem, this theory nevertheless shook the basis of physical and mathematical sciences in such measure that, notoriously, a tormented Einstein had to retort to an impassable Bohr: 'Do you really believe that God is playing dice with the world?', a remark intended to defend the existence of a well-coordinated, non-chaotic universe, a fundamental deterministic idea that Einstein's extraordinary intellect considered at the time as the most plausible. He could not, however, find respite for the rest of his career from attempting continuously to compile a comprehensive 'unified theory' connecting his 'theory of relativity' with the discoveries of quantum physics.

Unfortunately, he did not succeed in solving this all-important enigma during his lifetime. Moreover, regardless of recent advances in these domains, contemporary scientists present distinctive and often contradictory views on such issues as the origins of human life, the universe's evolution and the impact of quantum theory. They keep extending Einstein's work and attempt to align the major forces of nature, gravitational, nuclear and electromagnetic under one heading, possibly an all-embracing superforce. This 'theory of everything', however, still waits to be formulated reliably.

At the time of writing, Neil Turok Professor and Chair of Mathematical Physics at the University of Cambridge, announced the new theory he and Stephen Hawking had developed, concerning the beginnings of our universe. Starting from the idea of a Big Bang, a gigantic initial cosmic explosion secondary to which stars and galaxies were formed, they mathematically calculated that cosmic history may have started as an infinitesimal unique dot, a complex synthesis of time, space, matter and gravity, which subsequently exploded, inflated and continued to expand perpetually.

With its strong suggestion of a solitary, out-of-nothing, powerful commencement of the cosmos, the new discovery brought Professor Turok logically to the inescapable query of enormous general interest: 'Time to call for a creator?' Professor Turok admits that he does not believe in the existence of a divine force, nevertheless, the *New Scientist* in its October 1997 edition quoted a study demonstrating that 39.3 per cent of American scientists are convinced of the presence of a personal god to whom they usually direct their prayers.

The authors of the study, both from the University of Georgia at Athens, US remarked that while a relatively narrow definition of deity was used in their survey, it is possible that with a wider denomination, the proportion of believers would have been higher. Moreover, an interesting point is provided by the comparison with a 1916 survey of scientists, where 41.8 per cent voiced no doubt about the existence of a divine creator. There is, therefore, an almost unchanged attitude among the American scientific community.

The notion of a god that transcends time and space, brings into being 'something out of nothing', and whose basic forces master the workings of the cosmos, is not only a unifying factor among various religious traditions, but provides a focal point of safeguard for a human being as an individual. 'Do not cast me away in old age, when my strength gives out do not forsake me,' asks the psalmist (Psalms 71:9). The human condition, with its cohort of moral and physical suffering, finds in its connection with divinity an ideal means of releasing deep-seated fears, while invoking assistance in what often appear to be utterly hopeless situations.

Medical conditions are notoriously traumatising events, during which one's life is radically shaken. In moments of critical decision making, anger, apprehension and physical weakness, people commonly turn towards an exterior source of aid, fortuitously different from technological or pharmacological assistance. Although representing a subject that is only being emphasised in recent years, a majority of practicing physicians could, based on their experience, attest to the obvious influence played by belief and expectations in the shaping of the outcome of a disease.

To be discussed in more detail in the third part of the book, this subject provides an undeniable blueprint for the diagnostic and therapeutic domains of the future. The mystifying power of the human spirit will have to be taken into consideration as an integral part of the curative and restorative efforts, which in modern medicine include a long line of medications, interventional procedures and complementary remedies.

Einstein himself said in *Out of My Later Years*: 'It is only to the individual that a soul is given.' When calling upon faith, people appear to be able to gather all their emotional and mental resources, their inner driving force, subconsciously harboured and continuously striving for one's best. In the healing process, this can be transformed in an infallible impetus and a veritable lifeline for a patient facing a devastating physical problem.

The human soul, an indefinable entity that helps Man to carry the burden of his own mortality, appears suitably to fit the ancient Egyptian definition of the 'breath or essence of life'. In a certain sense, it has not only a self-assertive value, but also clear integrative capabilities, as it promotes a natural kinship between Man and the whole cycle of nature, with the latter viewed as a perennial, self-existent, dynamic and creative process.

> I am the plant of life
> Which comes forth from Osiris...
> Which allows the people to live
> Which makes the gods divine...
> Which enlivens the living,
> Which strengthens the limbs of the living.
> I live as corn, the life of the living...
> But the love of me is in the sky, on earth, on the water and in the fields...
> I am life appearing from Osiris.

At present, there is no distinct concept yet of the exact nature of life and, as such, not much seems to have changed since the times of the ancient Egyptians, as reflected in the above Coffin Text from the eighteenth dynasty, called 'Spell for Becoming Barley'. The benevolent god Osiris, symbolising cosmic origin, permanence and perpetual renewal, was often mentioned as the connector to a never-ending chain of life.

Modern Man, faced with different and, at the same time, astoundingly similar concerns, has the great challenge of using the advanced scientific discoveries of our era in order to augment his understanding of the miraculous workings of nature, including the enigmatic reality of the soul. This knowledge, when acquired, may represent a valuable and endless pool of vitality, a considerable source of comfort and growth for the years to come.

PART II

MESSAGES FROM THE PAST

Chapter 1

The Rod and the Fire

There was a time when meadow, grove, and stream,
The earth, and every common sight,
To me did seem
Apparelled in celestial light,
The glory and the freshness of a dream.

William Wordsworth,
Ode, Intimations of Immortality

The earliest times in mankind's history are usually viewed as eras of innocence, adaptation and discovery, part of a gradual and remarkable unfolding of human development. From utensils and artistic artefacts uncovered during archaeological excavations, much has been learned about the lives and customs of our most remote ancestors. This information is supplemented in great measure by observations made on the tribal communities of today, whose social organisation and cultural activities are considered to be equivalent to, or suggestive of, those exhibited by people living at the dawn of our civilisation.

Healing Connections

The Yoruba and Igbo of Nigeria, the Kung of North-East Kalahari, the Yanomamo of Venezuela and Brazil, the Australian Aborigines and the Native Americans all perpetuate rich, age-long traditions, full of an impressive artistic, ceremonial and functional content. Their wood, rock and cave paintings and carvings, inspirational music, and an extensive mythological lore demonstrate extraordinary insights into the workings of nature, as well as into essential human characteristics. The inner structure of a tribe can often be representative of the underlining life pattern of these people, centred on major survival issues, such as food gathering and distribution, childbirth and rearing, as well as defence against potential enemies.

In this context, a community leader has an important role to play, as he is required to channel the tribe's efforts towards a beneficial utilisation of natural resources and the development of peaceful, mutually supportive relationships between members of the clan. He or she is called upon to fulfil such varied functions as weather prediction, advice in matters of crop collection and animal breeding, mediation between belligerent parties and the organisation of festive ceremonies.

At the time of writing, elated newspapers report the striking performance achieved by two Yanomamo leaders who, by using ancestral prayers, seem to have brought much wanted rain over the burning Amazonian forest. They stopped what turned out to be one of the world's most horrendous ecological disasters. While succeeding where hundreds of firefighters, army helicopters and sophisticated weather-prediction devices could not, the indigenous wise men shed light yet again over the potential resources hidden in ancient traditions.

Possessors of a considerable amount of knowledge, often transmitted from father to son, chiefs of tribal communities around the world gain their repute based on decisions that are characterised by a deep concern for fellow tribesmen and

Messages from the Past

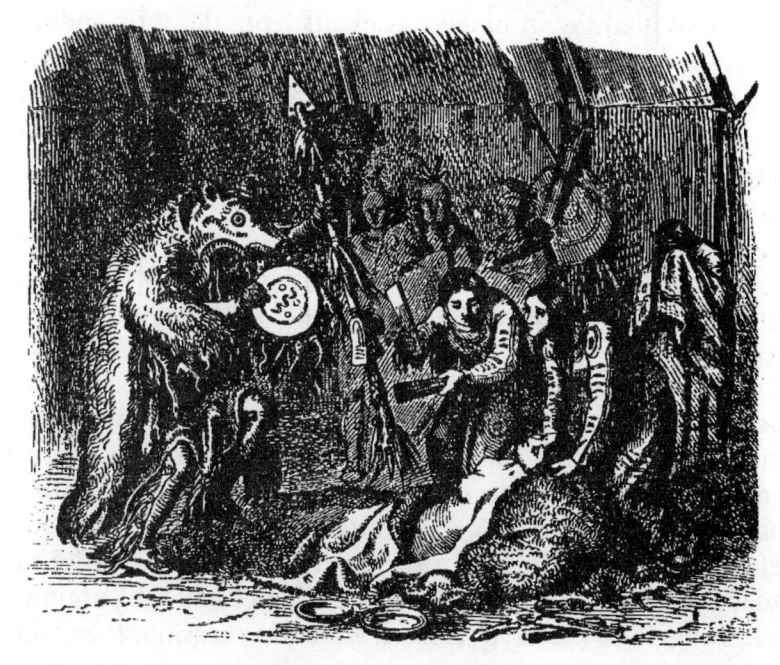

'Medicine Man' woodcut

women and affect all areas of life. None of these domains is more valued or more significant to the tribe's survival than the members' physical and emotional well-being. Thus being the leader of a native community will often mean also playing the role of medicine man (healer or shaman), a well-recognised function in the social organisation of many ancient and contemporary indigenous societies.

As intricate and daring as it may seem, the process of controlling people's health and supervising their behaviour in a world infested by micro- and macroscopic predators can be understood while grasping the unique role played by the tribesman's natural environment as an important source of inspiration, support and therapeutic means. For example, the medicinal qualities of numerous plants from the surrounding plains and forests were recognised early on by our ancestors, and used for the treatment of wounds and infections, broken bones, fever, skin rashes, abdominal pain and many other ailments. Numerous drugs belonging to the modern pharmacopoeia, such as curare (a powerful anesthetic), or reserpine (a common antihypertensive), have their origin in substances being used as long as hundreds of years ago by the Amazonian tribes, the Maya and the ancient people living in the Indian subcontinent.

As exemplified by modern tribal communities, the connection with Mother Nature implies an overwhelming willingness to comprehend 'the rules' governing the surrounding world and to live according to them. Shamen will attempt to interpret the hidden messages transmitted by the rainfall, the heat of the sun, the moonlight or the flowing river, and attempt to adapt them to the needs of human existence and the continuous struggle to preserve it. During a curing session, they will employ magical procedures meant to demonstrate the capability of mankind to interfere with the workings of nature and change their course, by a reconciliation of the human spirit with the perpetual universal force.

As much as this may signify a vision of the world involving a great deal of chance and uncoordinated circumstances, the tribal approach is entirely at odds with the theory of chaos. The cyclical movements of the stars and the planets, the perpetual return of the seasons and the ceaseless activity of the oceans and seas, continuously and attentively observed and admired, all seem to support the concept of a harmonious, well-organised universe in which Man occupies a privileged place.

The dramatic exhibition of a shaman's curing capabilities usually takes place during a communal gathering, while song, dance and magic are used to help involve elemental spirit forces alive in nature. An indigenous medicine man or woman may hold up a snake or a rod, representing the connection between the sky and the earth, the higher and lower realms, and he or she may choose to be near a burning fire or a pool of water, often seen as the symbols of infinite, preserving energy and the unconscious, hidden mysteries of the mind.

The notion of healing, therefore, is dealt with by native people in a manner that reflects a typical perception of reality, having to do mainly with the reinstatement of harmony and balance in a human life, and finding a way of doing so, by drawing the necessary energy from natural resources. As will be described in the next chapter, ancient Indian and Chinese medical traditions also deal significantly with the concept of energy or vital force. An example is the notion of the Kundalini movement, connecting various energy points in the body and taking place from the base of the spine to the brain, as well as the life energy *ch'i*, imbuing all living things, including humans, and providing the foundation for the functioning of all body parts.

It is thought that maintaining these energies and their proper flow ensures continuous health and a state of equilibrium in one's life. Therefore, when one equates energy with insight, determination, inner strength and adaptation capability, it is easy to comprehend why techniques directed towards the enhancement of this life force, such as acupuncture, martial arts or meditation, enjoy a worldwide following today.

Similarly, many tribal healers seem to have grasped the all-important concept of healing as a process of coordination, refinement and focusing, during which a wave of mental and emotional stimulation sustains the sufferer's failing resources and promotes a resurgence of its healing powers. This is extracted by the medicine man from his interaction with all creation, matter and spirit, viewed as one entity, a timeless and efficacious pool of vitality.

Healing Connections

My closest and earliest encounter with this candid and powerful identification with the natural world came from Florica ('Little Flower'), our maid of Romany origin. In my carefree childhood, under her supervision, recognising birds by their songs, climbing apple trees or leaping through the freezing waters of a mountain stream were enjoyable events and taken as natural occurrences. When Florica said, 'Smile, child, it will hurt less,' and treated my scraped knee with a plant remedy, it was all natural as well.

One day, a sudden gust of wind blew open the living-room window and the old woman said wistfully, 'It seems a king has passed away today.' Several minutes later, when my father entered the room and exclaimed, 'We have just heard horrible news: President Kennedy died!', I was glued to my chair with amazement and mumbled, 'Florica, how did you know...?' 'The spirit of the wind told me, honey,' she replied, simply.

I can remember experiencing a similar emotion when only five years old, listening to Brahms's first piano concerto played by Sviatoslav Richter, a magnificent pianist. The glorious, overwhelming opening impressed me immensely and gave a perplexing, vague and unmistakable sensation: that of a tangible presence of veiled realities.

Years later, as a physician with a strong interest in natural sciences, I developed a clearly Cartesian approach to medicine, including a distinctive need for rational analysis and the presence of facts to support my observations. The human body, studied in this manner, becomes a fascinating puzzle to be continuously unravelled. Its secret codes, as well as solutions to clinical problems, appear to be hidden in intricate chemical and physical formulae, the solving of which can eventually lead to the clarification of all biological processes. There are extraordinary traditions to be followed in the highly demanding world of scientific research, and much space for innovation, imagination and will, but the sphere of action remains firmly grounded, well documented and extremely suspicious of non-conforming, unverifiable issues.

The prevailing attitude of the scientific community is highly understandable. A long history of struggle against superstition and prejudice, with numerous heroes sacrificing their lives on the altar of freedom of thought and advancement of science, justifies the existent concern against unfounded theories and truth manipulations. During my entire career, I myself remained faithful to these principles, which I strongly attempted to combine with an unceasing curiosity and an open mind.

While pursuing my other interest, the study of ancient civilisations and their medical traditions, I also perceived the great need to reconcile the old with the new, the modern with the traditional, to reunite under one roof modalities that are basically directed towards the same valuable service, the improvement of humanity's existence.

A world of differences separates the two approaches, exemplified firstly by linguistic inadequacies, related mainly to the meaning of various criteria and expressed opinions. It is almost impossible to define scientifically what an Amerindian means when he says: 'the power of your dream', 'the measure of your soul' or 'wholeness of heart'. Concepts such as energy, stillness, movement, life, death, getting better or succeeding, differ greatly among the traditional and the modern, mainly due to the fact that the Western linguistic system is based on static definitions, while native idioms include the significant presence of movement, dynamism, cyclical change and transformation. In this sense, being healed, for example, does not mean necessarily getting rid of a body defect, but recovering from emotional and physical malaise, readjusting to the increasing demands of one's body and learning how to function anew. Bridging the gap between modern medical techniques and ancient healing traditions requires the recognition of an intricate system of relationships connecting the healer to the healed, to the drugs provided, to their specific mode of administration, as well as to the timing and inner rhythm of the healing process. The whole, uninterrupted flow finds its conducive strength in the natural, universal store of energy, to which both the healer and the patient have access through their relentless efforts.

It is well known that a great majority of native medicine men and women must reach a state of altered consciousness in order to perform a curing ceremony successfully. Nevertheless, even in this domain, a common denominator can be found between them and successful Western-style physicians, as they are both animated by the same dedication to the task and high ethical values. Indeed, it can be demonstrated that although numerous people have, by various techniques, mastered the ability to change at will the level of their consciousness, rare are those able to interfere and positively influence the course of a disease process. Evidently, such a proficiency requires a complete immersion into an assignment, which very much becomes a labour of generosity and care.

Some time ago, during a social gathering, I met a renowned psychic who told me that he was never involved in healing. The person before me seemed agitated, vociferous and self-centred, and I immediately understood the reason for his stance. Undoubtedly, the power plug of a successful medical therapy lies in the human qualities of both the giver and the receiver of the treatment, in their acceptance of a bond of confidence and togetherness, creating in the patient of a suitable mental and emotional status and overcoming the inherent difficulties related to recovery from illness.

Can, therefore, ancient healing traditions provide some additional and useful insights into the workings of the human psyche and its influence on the physiological functioning of the body? The answer is most certainly yes, especially as they imply an active patient participation and his sharing the responsibility of getting better. In modern psychological studies there is no proper classification for the type of activity performed by a shaman. Although numerous tomes have been dedicated to the subject, the array of customs and symbols, including sensory and physical deprivation, fasting, ritual chanting and dancing, as well as the use of sacred 'medicines' (plants, pebbles, feathers, etc.), is still considered as belonging to the borderline realm of the 'paranormal', to which, despite numerous attempts, there are currently not enough examples of any biochemical or neurophysiological relationships available.

Anthropologists studying the way of life of the Kung of Kalahari, the Alaskan and Siberian Eskimos and the North American Indians, among many other tribal communities where shamanic activities are common, have recognised the pertinent differences between Western-type language and mentality and tribal societies' culture. Pertinent to this book's subject, the holistic approach in the area of physical disease alleviation is only one facet of the kaleidoscope of native practices covering all essential life domains, such as farming, hunting, getting married or going to war.

When attempting to translate fitting indigenous expressions accurately, existent vocabulary and conceptual barriers prevent us from obtaining the global picture, that of a highly integrated system with a strong and characteristic belief structure concerning the nature of illness and health. The personal and social implications of becoming sick are always recognised in the light of the purpose of life as understood by the native. The gravest occurrence of all is not to die, as death is seen as merely a phase in a perpetual existence, but to lose one's capability of being part of the whole, of all living and non-living things on earth and in the skies.

The purpose of much shamanic healing is therefore directed firstly towards restoring the lost emotional balance resulting from being excluded, being different. The extended ceremonies, often enjoying the entire tribe, augment a sense of belonging, of companionship and have a substantial influence on the moral strengthening of the ill. Injury or infections are dealt with only in the second instance, the first step being dedicated to the enforcement of the individual, to the return of his or her confidence and self-reliance.

As mentioned before, incorrect translations have until now perpetuated numerous misunderstandings, supported in part by the healing rituals that, when observed by the learned researcher, seem complicated and strange enough to deter him or her from interpreting in greater depth their essential significance. Still, if better analysed, shamanic practices appear to parallel new medical findings, which show that in order to improve our success at treating illness, a more unified and general therapeutic approach is necessary.

What is recognised when dealing with psychosomatic disorders and an increasing number of other illnesses that have such a developed psychological component, is that the modern physician, much as the shaman with his 'ancient way', will need firstly to balance the patient's mind, so that out of emotional and mental chaos healing can begin. While for a scientifically educated practitioner it is easy to visualise the human body as a universe of chemical and physical energies, the presence of spiritual energy is not something immediately apparent or acceptable.

From this point of view, the modern physician and the native medicine man have different 'objects' to practise on. The latter's patient is born with the conviction that a human life is not worth living unless the soul is preserved. This notion encompasses the capability of integration into the endless web of life, of resilience and permanence, and certainly has a wider significance than the one generally accepted by Western philosophies.

When unwell, a native will place his fate with complete trust into the hands of his healer, who quite often endures horrendous initiation trials and demonstrates extraordinary stamina for performances that can last from days to weeks. The cooperation between the sick and the shaman are at a level at which the degree of expectancy is exceptionally high and inner conflicts are smoothed out. This undoubtedly influences the outcome of the treatment.

There is certainly a need to appreciate shamanic medicine realistically, without any attempt to glamorise it. Difficulties encountered by some tribal communities are well known and include high infant mortality due to birth trauma or infections, gastro-intestinal disorders resulting from improper water or food resources, parasitic infestations, malnutrition and low life expectancy. Nevertheless, Western medical practitioners can certainly benefit from the information provided by the natives' experiences and their intuitive perception of the healing process.

Learning from the shaman and using certain aspects of his approach is not easy, as it requires the preparation of both the patient and the physician for a closer interaction, and a more detailed appreciation of a physical imbalance. Recognising the fact that human physiology is greatly influenced by psychological fluctuations, medical intervention should be directed mainly towards those factors that take the patient 'out of synchronicity with his or her normal rhythm', reinstalling mental and emotional peace, an ideal background for healing. This approach coincides with the native's awe and wonder for the workings of the human body and his devout humility before the harmony of nature.

Chapter 2

Healing Rivers

Do we build houses for ever?
Does the river for ever rise up and brings on floods?
The dragon-fly leaves its shell
That its face may but glance at the face of the sun.
Since the days of yore there has been no permanence.

The Epic of Gilgamesh

The year is 1765 BC. We stroll through one of the many souks serving the famous city of Babylon. Its Akkadian name, *Bâb-ilâni* (the Gate of the Gods), fittingly depicts a rich and powerful capital, whose palaces, libraries and gardens are unmatched in size and beauty. Busy, well-dressed people move about, buying, selling and discussing the main issues of the day.

In the midst of the many-tongued bustle, an unusual scene is attracting our attention. A frail, old man, lying on a carpet on the ground, is surrounded by a group of individuals, each of them appearing to discuss with him matters of great impor-

Messages from the Past

tance. We are told that the old man is ill and people around him are well-wishers who, based on their knowledge and personal experience, attempt to offer counsel.

Herodotus, the famous Greek historian (485–425 BC), described the custom: 'In Babylon the entire nation is the physician. They bring out their sick to the market place, then those who pass by the sick person confer with him about the disease and advise him to have recourse to the same treatment as that by which they escaped a similar ailment, or as they have known to cure others. None may pass by the sick man without speaking and asking what his sickness is.'

Clearly, the inhabitants of the ancient land bordered by the Tigris and Euphrates rivers were not relying solely on the *asu* (the specialised physician) to decide on matters of health and disease. As described by Herodotus, they approached medical issues in a manner that exemplified a generalised and well-informed concern.

Builders of an astoundingly developed culture, justifiably named 'the cradle of civilisation', Sumerians, Akkadians and, later on, Assyrians and Babylonians, demonstrated a rare insight into the workings of the human body. In a well-developed scientific environment, unprecedented progress was made in various domains, including mathematics, astronomy, metallurgy, architecture and law.

Hammurabi, a powerful king of Babylon thought to have reigned between 1792 and 1750 BC, codified medical activities and established strict conduct regulations. These included severe punishments for medical 'errors' and appropriate remuneration for dedicated healers. His 'code of law' can still be admired, engraved on a black diorite column preserved at the Louvre Museum in Paris.

In general, Mesopotamian culture demonstrated an original and sophisticated approach to human health, as registered

Healing Connections

on thousands of clay tablets inscribed in the advanced and elegant cuneiform writing. By developing a system of thought centred around the great mysteries of life, ancient Mesopotamians refined existent knowledge and attempted to obtain a reply to fundamental human uncertainties, such as the place of Man in the grand scheme of the universe, and the cause of calamities afflicting mankind, including of illness.

A healer of that time, close to our concept of a modern physician, employed drugs to treat his patients and performed surgical interventions. But mainly he worked on establishing a full and correct patient history. This was based not only on information gathered on past illnesses, present complaints and diseases encountered in the patient's family, but on an accurate analysis of the patient's mental state, including a detailed account of his dreams. Such a remarkable approach predated by many centuries the modern tendency towards viewing organic and psychological disturbances as closely related.

Highly knowledgeable about the movements of the stars and the appearance of comets, ancient Mesopotamians were fully aware of the existence of a powerful and crucial mind-body connection. They based their medical observations on anatomical sections of body organs and were able to diagnose accurately the extent of a disease process. At the same time, their rare comprehension of the workings of the human psyche greatly influenced their medical conclusions.

Carrying an unmistakable 'flavour', healing practices of the time were the result of an intriguing mixture of superstitious beliefs and a realistic interpretation of the functioning of the human body. Accordingly, a large number of omens were taken into consideration when examining a patient, as disparate as the direction of the wind, the colours of the surrounding area, or the presence or absence of river flooding. In

Messages from the Past

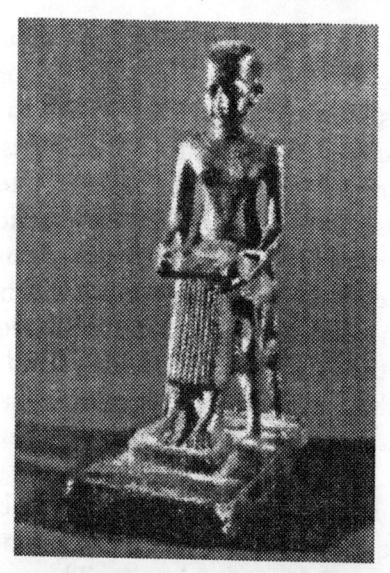

Imhotep, Egyptian architect and physician, advisor to Pharoah Djoser

addition, evil spirits and demons were considered to be propagators of diseases, while ritual incantations were specially composed for the purpose of chasing them away.

These prayerful invocations were recited during curing ceremonies, which employed sound and rhythm to create a vibrational harmony able to induce mental relaxation and enhance the therapeutic effect of the various drugs used. In this sense, mystical Mesopotamian doctrines can be perceived as promoters of a state of spiritual attunement, intimately connected to the act of healing.

On the more pragmatic side, as mentioned before, decisions on the type of treatment to be administered would always include a rigorous analysis of the psychological makeup of each individual. This relied heavily on the assumption that the major cause for illness was to be found in the breakdown of the precious and fragile inner balance, essential for an organism's satisfactory function. The healer's main effort, directed towards the reinstatement of this lost equilibrium, represented the guiding principle in the therapeutic process.

King Ashurbanipal's famous library, excavated at the site of the beautiful Assyrian capital Nineveh, provided invaluable information on how medicine was practised around 600 BC. Greatly influenced by religion, the local inhabitants respectfully followed the directives received from a rich pantheon of gods, including the creator-gods An, Enlil and Enki, the sun-god Shamash, the goddess of love Ishtar (Inanna), and the mother-goddess Ninhursag, creator of numerous healing deities.

The forces in heaven, considered to have absolute control over the world, dictated its rules and in great measure impregnated the course of human history. This concept is well reflected in the fabulous myths and tales that this prodigious civilisation left with us, and which comprise among others, stories related to the creation of the universe, the occurrence of the flood and the existence of the tower of Babel.

However, as demonstrated in the renowned *Epic of Gilgamesh*, Sumerians, Babylonians and Assyrians were constantly challenging their divine masters, searching for answers to humanity's most ardent quests: the nature of human life and death, the principle of destiny and the eternal cosmic struggle between good and evil. Precisely in the same manner in which the forces of chaos were able at any moment to attack and destroy the well-established order on earth, physical and mental illnesses were viewed as intruders that disrupted the mental and physiological status quo, without which normal functioning of the human body was not possible.

According to legend, the hero Gilgamesh, absorbed by his willingness to live for ever, was rebuked by the gods and found understanding only with Utnapishtim, the man elected by the gods to survive the flood and granted eternal life. 'Do not search for immortality,' Utnapishtim advised the young king, 'it is reserved for the mighty deities in the sky. The ability to remain healthy and live a happy life lies within yourself.'

In other words, the promoted concept was to chase away the tendency to look for external help and to develop one's inner ability to confront and overcome adversity, including illness and the process of ageing. Gilgamesh understood the message and returned to the capital Uruk, where he reigned for many years as a powerful and content king.

We sense from the tale the intriguing capability of ancient Mesopotamians to grasp the inestimable value of willpower, self-control and relaxation in the successful management of human life. This aspect is also prominently featured in the mythical healing tradition of the ancient land of Egypt, inhabited as early as five to six millennia ago:

> The One the sister without equal,
> The most beautiful of all,
> She resembles the rising morning star,
> At the beginning of a happy year.
> Shining bright, fair of skin,
>
> Lovely the look of her eyes,
> Sweet the speech of her lips...
> True lapis-lazuli her hair,
> Her arms surpassing gold...
>
> (Papyrus Chester Beatty I: Verso)

The goddess Hathor-Sekhmet, praised in this poem by faithful followers, provided the necessary focus for the establishment of numerous places of worship in ancient Egypt. In these temples, specialised priests acted as religious guides, as well as reliable medical practitioners. These were times in which belief in the power of the supernatural represented a constant component of the healing art.

Medical teachings revolved, therefore, around a great number of healing deities, such as Thoth, the ibis or baboon-headed god of knowledge; Isis, the mother goddess, often invoked for protection and cure, and Imhotep, the son of the venerated god Ptah, living at the time of King Djoser (third dynasty, c 2686–2613 BC). A remarkable healer, the latter was to become the centre of a veritable cult, where the patient was at the core of its concerns.

It would thus be greatly unjustified to view the use by this civilisation of magic incantations, spells and sacred rituals as merely delusive techniques aimed to enhance popular reliance on powerful gods. As recorded in a great number of medical papyri (the Ebers, the Kahun, the Edwin Smith, and many others), besides a large variety of natural products offered as sophisticated medical prescriptions, sick people in ancient Egypt were treated in an atmosphere of tranquility and spiritual exaltation, recognised as being capable of considerably reinforcing the effect of the recommended 'pharmacological' treatment.

Moreover, patient isolation in calm surroundings was achieved by the construction of sanatoria (healing houses), dedicated to the care of the sick. The Ptolemaic temple of the goddess Hathor at Deidra serves as a good example of such a specialised compound. There, in small cubicles surrounding a body of water, and in the neighbourhood of a temple dedicated to a major healing deity, patients would spend their nights hoping to have a revelatory dream. Its contents could prove capable of identifying the reasons for their malaise, as well as proposing a suitable cure. Dream interpretation and immersion in holy water formed the basis for a comprehensive assessment of an individual's state, a combination of magical beliefs and the very realistic insight that 'what is on one's mind' may represent a clue to his or her illness.

The word *swnw* (soo-noo or suenew) designated a physician or a doctor of the time practising conventional medicine. The name was often preceded by a hierarchical title or followed by a denomination related to his specialisation, such as *swnw irty* (ophthalmologist), *swnw khat* (gastroenterologist), and so on. Interestingly enough, the sentence 'placing the hand', which appears so often in the Egyptian medical documents of that era, reflects most probably one of the principal ways in which a physician examined, communicated with, or treated the patient. The symbol exemplifies well the pursuit of a very close doctor–patient relationship, as well as the existence of a climate of quietude, trust and introspection, instrumental for the achievement of a cure.

A similar outlook became the signpost of a civilisation developing along the Indus valley from around 1500 BC. The oldest scriptures of Hinduism belong to these nomadic Aryan people, who came from the north to inhabit the Indian subcontinent. Named *Vedas* ('divine knowledge' in Sanskrit), they embodied the collective lore of the time, in the form of hymns, chants, prayers and sacrificial formulae.

Ayurveda the traditional Indian system of medicine, was based on principles derived from the *Vedas* and represented, as its name attests (literally 'knowledge of life'), a doctrine aimed better understanding the rules governing the universal order, as well as developing behaviour patterns capable of ensuring an uneventful integration of human life into it. Apart from a religious content, medical advice and proposed treatments related to general health, the essential component of

Indian medical teachings was made up of innovative suggestions for mind-control techniques.

As emphasised by the prevailing philosophical doctrines, the human self had the task of unifying itself with the cosmic, universal spirit. Metaphysical and ethical precepts were invoked in order to support this eternal quest and justify the belief in the transmigration of souls. Consequently, humans were requested to live up to standards of piety, goodness and justice, enabling the acquisition of a suitable *karma*. *Karma* was believed to follow a soul through its successive rebirths, from one generation to another, until the time when a favourable past *karma* resulted in a state of grace and a complete fusion with the universal power.

The vicissitudes of daily life, the Hindus considered, generally restricted humans from achieving the mental and physical states required by the holy scriptures. They therefore developed several methods for reneging the 'bodily pleasures in life', doing away with desire and concentrating on spiritual knowledge. Even if much of Western society today finds it difficult to identify with the ideals of spiritual and physical purity propagated by Hindu teachings, it is obvious that many of their basic practices have found a large following.

A perfect representative of these behavioural tactics, the doctrine of yoga ('union' in Sanskrit), was initially directed towards a mystical fusion with the divine, through a regimen of meditation, adoption of special postures and ascetic practices. Introduced to the West in the late nineteenth century, yoga became enormously popular, because of its capacity to lead to a state of mental concentration able to control nerve centres and internal vital forces.

Modern therapeutic techniques have adopted yoga as a reliable method of inducing relaxation and alleviating stress.

Meditation, an important component of the same philosophical system and usually linked to various religious practices (in Hindu and other cultures), has been associated in recent years with fitness programmes, including yoga, and alternative or complementary medical therapies.

Medical studies can show that the usage of the above practices is entirely justified, as changes in body metabolism occurring during meditation and controlled physical exercise include a reduction in blood pressure, a slowing of the pulse rate and increased vascular circulation to the periphery. By freeing the mind from rigid conscious control, yoga and meditation help an individual to let go and function successfully according to the deeper and quieter layers of his or her self.

Related to the same approach, visualisation was utilised in the Hindu tradition as a process during which the mind's eye was trained to construct images capable of enhancing physical and mental healing. It is not surprising, therefore, that activating one's imagination or guiding one's positive fantasies has developed into an important modern clinical tool. As an aid to medication and conventional therapies, it is currently used in numerous medical centres around the globe and proves highly efficient in the treatment of numerous conditions, including heart disease, psychosomatic disorders, cancers and trauma.

Additionally, mandalas, pictorial symbols of the universe drawn by Buddhist monks, and employed in the meditative process, demonstrate well the main goal advocated by this ancient tradition, that of a continuous search for inner peace and harmony. Much of the psychological concepts were developed by the Swiss neurologist Carl Gustav Jung, who took further this idea and viewed mandalas as reflections of the self, with a close correspondence between the symmetry of the image and the wholeness of the psychological makeup of an individual.

With time, principles of Ayurvedic medicine were transmitted to neighbouring China, the vast land traversed by the Yellow River. Meditation, breathing techniques, gymnastics and yoga became, by AD 700, an integral part of Chinese medical practices. These influences, however, did not reach a cultural vacuum. On the contrary, as early as 3000 BC, medicine was fully developed in China, with eminent representatives, such as the Yellow Emperor, Huang Ti, who wrote the impressive *Nei Ching*, the Canon of Medicine.

Aside from innovative medical advice, this tome included extensive psychological guidance to be used in a great variety of maladies. Most of it was based on the existence of the fundamental principles of Yin and Yang, which together with the five elements (earth, water, iron, wood and metal), ruled everything in the universe and formed life's tangible essence.

In this concept, positive, dark, male and evolutionary fractions found themselves to be in combination with negative, bright and female constituents, in order to support the vital laws of unification and to contribute to the formation of the all-important *ch'i*. This energy force, thought to control the functioning of the entire human body, had to be sustained, nourished and preserved from annihilation by adopting a golden, healthy way.

> The greatest virtues come only from the Tao, their source...
> The forms of all things crouch within it
> Eluding touch and sight...
> Only the semblance of all things remains.
> The Tao is profound dark and obscure;
> The essence of all things endures there.

Around the year 600 BC, a contemporary of Confucius, named Lao Tzu, compiled a book of precepts entitled *The Tao Te Ching* (the Canon of Reason and Virtue), from which these verses are taken. Essentially it summarised the fundamental belief of that time, that Man represented merely a small component of a vast, complex and still largely unknown system, in which every element, even the most minuscule, had its importance.

Drawing on powerful images and symbols, the text provides a typical example of how the ancient Chinese thought to achieve a harmonious integration of human life both into surrounding nature and the demanding social organisation. 'Follow the Tao,' was the advice. That is, embrace a behavioural pattern that will allow you to gain a state of mental and emotional peace, closely resembling the mechanics of God's universe, where everything acts in an enduring unity.

Medical art in ancient China surrendered entirely to the spiritual and philosophical atmosphere embodied in the *Tao Te Ching*. This was clearly reflected in specialised medical treatises, such as the Yellow Emperor's *Nei Ching*, mentioned before, or the works of two other mythical 'gods' of medicine, Fu Hsi, the Celestial Emperor and Shen Nung, the Fire Emperor.

As pictured in these compilations, Chinese medical tradition seemed to sustain, more than any other ancient doctrine, a most convincing vision of the human organism working as one unit, as well as of the powerful influence exerted by the hidden mental resources of each individual in preserving this wholeness. Renowned Chinese therapeutic techniques, such as acupuncture (the insertion of needles along specific body meridians, believed to transmit the life force *ch'i*) or moxibustion (the excitation of various skin trigger points by burning a powdered plant substance), followed the same basic principle of treating the human organism as an integral entity.

Moreover, the value of an intuitive approach to a patient's problems has been stressed continuously as the ultimate means of arriving at a correct diagnosis. The majority of ancient Chinese written material, including the famous *I Ching* (a reliable oracle whose answers were said to never fail), seems to promote a refined technique for using of the subconscious mind, with the enquirer being guided by his inner, unmediated perception to find the best solution to a problem. A Chinese healer was therefore strongly persuaded to develop this unique and valuable insight before beginning to provide help.

A veritable amalgam of concepts and practices, Chinese medical methodology also included the views promoted by Kung Fu-tzu, the famous Confucius, who lived between 550 and 479 BC. Without excluding the possibility of a spiritual power governing the world, Confucius focused mainly on paying tribute to life's realities, while praising the essential, centrally located human being, who was perceived as a superior creature, capable of controlling both his body and his environment and deciding on his or her own fate.

External factors were considered by the ancient Chinese to be able to influence heavily the health balance of an individual. Problems usually occurred when too much (*tai-kuo*) or too little (*pu-chi*) was offered. On the other hand, a patient himself, aided by his healer, could exert just the right control (*cheng*) over his life, by selecting the appropriate mental attitude, and, not only to correct any occurring imbalances, but also to avert most of the time the prospect of becoming ill.

From the ancient approaches to the principle of *mens sana in corpore sano* (a healthy mind in a healthy body), professed by the Roman satirist Juvenal around the year AD 60, is merely one historical step. These astonishing early ancient civilisations with their impressive codes of personal and social behaviour exerted a profound influence on subsequent Greek and Roman antiquity. Their comprehensive and world-changing medical doctrines will be reviewed in the next chapter.

Chapter 3

The Giant of Kos

The gods help those who help themselves.
Aesop, *Fables*, 'Hercules and the Wagoner'

Athena, the virgin goddess of war, intelligence and wisdom sprang full-grown and armoured from the head of her father, Zeus. The ancient Greeks worshipped and feared her, while building magnificent temples in her honour, such as the Parthenon in Athens, the impressive ruins of which can still be admired today. The city itself was named after the beloved goddess, in recognition for her gift of an olive tree to the local people.

An active participant in numerous battles, such as the renowned Trojan War, she was followed by young Greeks who had the chance to prove their prodigious vigour, acquired as a result of the well-organised system of physical education in ancient Greece. From early childhood, the practice of sports such as foot races, wrestling, spear and disc throwing, and boxing, were strongly encouraged.

Among the chief goals to be attained was the harmonious development of the body, accompanied by an unrivalled endurance of pain and fatigue. The importance of such strenuous athletic training lay in its capability to influence the intellectual and moral qualities of an individual.

Grace, ease of bearing and strength of character were considered paramount features of a person successfully integrated into ancient Greek society. These attributes were supposed to protect one from laziness, corruption and selfishness, and to model individuals into useful and well-adjusted citizens. The arts of the time – numerous sculptures, mosaics, frescoes and vase paintings, containing exquisite and eloquent representations of human figures, both male and female – reflect this search for perfection of the body.

The largest number of participants at the Hellenic sport competitions were men who regularly worked out in magnificent gymnasiums (*gymnos*, naked). However, women were also encouraged to take great care of their bodies and, indeed, actively participated in athletic contests, mainly in gymnastic exercises. In general, young people joining the ancient Greek cycles of games (the Olympics being the most famous), were elected from the general population rather than professional athletes. Transformed into grandiose public spectacles, usually involving prolonged feasts and the performance of music and dances, the sports competitions of the time greatly contributed to enhancing the appreciation of physical beauty as an inherent companion of high moral standards.

This attitude can be traced back to the underlining philosophical concepts that characterised an epoch of unmatched cultural and scientific developments. Socrates (*c.* 469 to *c.* 399 BC), his pupil Plato (*c.* 428 to *c.* 347 BC) and the latter's student, Aristotle (384–322 BC) were the most illustrious representatives of the period's relentless search for knowledge and truth, with special emphasis placed on the study of human existence, viewed always in comparison with other living things, such as plants and animals.

In some of the most influential writings in the history of thought, Plato and Aristotle opened the road for a better understanding of the workings of the universe, the ways in which mankind could survive in the midst of surrounding nature and adjust to the requirements of social life. Medicine of the time became an integral part of this generalised trend, despite the continuous belief in the influence of immortal Olympian gods on all aspects of human life, including matters of illness and health. The revered deities were considered capable of establishing intricate relationships with people, advising and supporting them, while at the same time inflicting severe punishments for unacceptable behaviour, such as arrogance, selfishness or exaggerated ambitions.

Among the worshipped gods and goddesses, the main ones considered responsible for health matters were Apollo, upon whom were bestowed important curing capabilities (he was described by Homer as playing physician to the gods), and the mythical healer Asklepios who, according to legend, was Apollo's son. Asklepios can be easily identified with Imhotep, the venerated Egyptian god of medicine, whose traditions he was clearly continuing.

As with their counterparts in ancient Egypt, numerous healing centres developed in the Greek islands, some of them becoming notorious for their size and lavishness, such as the sanctuaries of Epidauros, Athens and Pergamon. Here, the same distinguishing features could be found, attesting for a system of medical therapy based on patient relaxation and purification. These ancient spas always included a spring of fresh water (*thalos*), a pool in which people could bathe, and a stadium for the performance of physical exercise, all components of an environment designed to instil a feeling of well-being and separation from harmful agents.

The presence of sophisticated sleeping quarters contributed also to the creation of an atmosphere of peace and confidence, in which patients could release their fears and express their innermost hopes. This was the place were the healer visited the ill, talked to and consulted them individually and applied the necessary remedies. Similar to the custom in ancient Egypt and Mesopotamia, the dreams of the patients were analysed, as they were considered to reflect the psychological state of the patient, a factor that greatly influenced the existence of diseases, as well as the ability to conquer them.

Against this inspirational background, scientific medicine emerged as an inherent branch of philosophy, which at the time attempted to provide rational, rather than mystical, explanations for natural events, including the functioning of the human body. The Ancient Greek physicians, named *iatros*, continued to believe in the existence of healing gods, but at the same time strove to understand the structure of body organs and how to improve their workings when necessary.

Preceded by a long list of eminent philosophers–scientists such as Thales of Miletus, Anaximender, Empedocles and Pythagoras, Hippocrates, the 'father of medicine', was born, according to tradition, in 460 BC on the island of Kos, near the coast of Asia Minor. While establishing a renowned medical and philosophical school on the island, his efforts and those of other physicians from parallel medical schools, such as the one in the neighbouring city of Cnidon, resulted in a large number of advanced and important medical principles that form the basis of the Western therapeutic system today.

It is certainly important to mention the successful manner

in which these ancient physicians, writers of exceptional medical works, combined scientific work with seriousness, modesty, purity of life and, most importantly, a medical approach in which Man and his best interests were at the centre of attention. While considering that a vital force, the *thymos*, supplied humans with vigour during their lifetimes and left them at death, they generally agreed in the simultaneous existence of a timeless component to human life; *psyche*, the soul. Consequently, the physical and mental preparation prior to treatment had strong spiritual undertones, aiming to strengthen the patient's faith in the healer's efforts and the efficacy of the treatment.

At that time mathematical principles and powerful doctrines, based on the influence of numbers in nature, made for a wide distribution of Pythagoras's views on the existence of cosmic order and harmony. According to this theory, there was a mathematical basis to the universe attesting for its perpetuity and therefore humans were advised to behave according to its governing rules, and set their 'inner clocks' in concordance with the famous 'harmony of the spheres', i.e. the intricate and instrumental relationship between the movement of celestial bodies, numbers, music and human destiny.

'What we have to learn to do, we learn by doing,' said Aristotle in his *Metaphysics*. Mentions can therefore be found in the medical literature of the time on how to achieve continuous health by pursuing a regimen of a vegetarian diet, gymnastics, music and meditation and, in general, by attempting to bring a degree of perfection to daily life. The notion of *isonomia*, introduced by Alcmaeon of Crotona, a pupil of Pythagoras, emphasised the absolute agreement in which all body elements coexist. Medical precepts connected in this manner important anatomical discoveries with recommendations for personal hygiene, behaviour during times of health crisis and the use of nature's harmonic ability to heal.

Hippocrates is known to have composed an oath, still in use today by medical practitioners. It contains moral and social guidelines for the healing profession, demonstrating the high ethical standards of the era. Based on irreproachable requirements and highest standards of devotion and reliability in the care of the ill, it has a timeless and considerable educational value, easily adaptable to modern conditions.

Ancient Greek physicians clearly continued an unbroken chain of medical practices that let compassion, sympathy and understanding play first fiddle in medical diagnosis and treatment. This tradition attached substantial importance to the deeper, more personal and emotional side of human nature and, with this, hinted at the available curing possibilities existing within this vast and powerful domain.

Incorporating the above Hellenistic principles, the Roman Empire combined the use of magical healing procedures with newly discovered drugs of vegetable and mineral origin, and saw a continuation, at least in the first centuries of our era, of the development of numerous sciences, including biology, history, medicine and geography. Prominent authorities of the time such as Cato, Varro, Pliny the Elder and Celsus were accomplished scientists, excelling in numerous fields of study. In the medical domain, the most renowned was the Roman physician of Greek origin, Galen (AD *c.* 129 to *c.* 200), one of antiquity's most prolific and influential compilers of books.

His ideas reverberated well into the Middle Ages, carrying with them the imprint of an original and dedicated thinker with extensive practical experience, resulting from his function as physician to the gladiators. Caring for seriously injured people and needing to support them physically and morally provided enough material for Galen to appreciate the great importance of willpower, stamina and self-preservation in situations when mere survival is at stake.

His study of the human character resulted in a classification that followed the physiological beliefs of the time, based on the presence of four body humours: phlegm, blood, chyle and bile. The description of the four personality types thus emerged; the phlegmatic, the sanguine, the choleric and the melancholic. It soon became obvious that the prevalence of certain diseases and, indeed, responses to treatment were strongly connected to the psychological makeup of an individual.

Typical in this regard is the discordance expressed by Galen with the views of some physicians such as Asklepiades (*c.* 120–70 BC), who wanted to cure *tuto, celerites ac jucunde* (safely, quickly and pleasantly), and considered that nature and the patient have nothing to do with diseases, the doctor's decisions playing the major role in the healing process.

The Romans continued to promote hygiene, nutrition and physical education, although their times were characterised by excesses in the latter domains, competitive games being often pushed to the level of fighting until death, while proverbial feasts were described as involving unlimited eating and drinking. A prevailing promotion of corporeal pampering and search for mental relaxation is attested also by the presence of famous recreation centres (balnea or thermae), which flourished on the ancient Italian peninsula. In an atmosphere of indulgence and of searching for momentary enjoyment, Roman poets, writers and philosophers supported the view expressed by the Carthagian born dramatist, Terence: *Homo sum; humani nihil a me alienum puto* (I am a man; and nothing human is foreign to me).

They describe in their works a society greatly interested in going through the widest range of human experiences or, in the words of the playwright Seneca (c. 4 BC to c. 65 AD): 'As long as you live, learn how to live.' (*Epistulae ad Lucilium*) Conquering disease and suffering was an important aspect of personal development and was supposed to be handled by the Roman healer in close cooperation with the patient. 'Place the question to the patient himself,' advocated Emperor Trajan's physician, Rufus of Ephesus in *On Interrogation of the Patient*, 'as in this way you can learn if his mind is healthy, or otherwise, and get an idea on the disease he is suffering.'

Under the influence of Aristotle's teachings, Galen developed an interesting philosophical concept that had important repercussions in the medical area. He stated that nothing in nature was superfluous and the best way for mankind to understand God's purposes was by examining the workings of nature. As a result, his observations on the structure of the human body, which he saw as an integral part of the universal matrix, were intimately connected to the search for the best ways of improving its functioning.

'The universe is change; life is what thinking makes of it.' (*Meditations, IV*) The words of the Stoic philosopher Marcus Aurelius (AD 121–180) delineate an intellectual dilemma in which much space was given to personal initiative and determination. All things, he believed, 'come from eternity, are of similar forms and come around in a circle' (*Meditations, II*). At the same time, he understood that people could play an important role in designing their own destinies and pursuing specific goals, such as the attainment of physical and mental health. While fighting the various factors attempting to undermine their ability to do so, being in the right 'state of mind' represented a decisive constituent and a faithful ally. 'You should pray for a healthy mind in a healthy body,' advised his older contemporary, the satirist Juvenal in *Satires, X*.

And, as any other fun-loving Roman, he would undoubtedly have added, '*et permitte divis cetera*' (and leave the rest to the gods).

Chapter 4

In Tune with Eternity

We feel and we know that we are eternal.

Baruch Spinoza, *Ethics*

I was in Cannes for a medical congress and met Anthony R. while searching for a free table in an overcrowded sidewalk café, full of noisy holidaymakers. We had not seen each other for several years and immediately exchanged information on our personal and professional lives. I was really glad to meet him. Being a professional diplomat, Anthony travelled the world and was recognised as a refined and knowledgeable collector of folkloric art. He also studied history and comparative religion, and as such made a wonderful conversation partner.

Anthony was, I soon found out, recovering from a serious disease. In his words, 'It almost put an end to my life, worse yet, my sanity...' While apologising for succumbing to the unfortunate habit people often have, that of discussing their health problems with every physician they meet, he told me the story of his brief but horrendous battle with weakness, pain and incapacitation, ending in a victory against all odds.

Later on, we walked along the boardwalk The sea was shimmering under the setting sun and a pleasant breeze was slowly dispersing the day's heat. The decorum went well with the subject at heart. We talked about peace.

'The most difficult thing to do,' said Anthony, 'was to let go of old habits and grasp the need to tap into powers as infinite as the sea before us, the most hidden resources within oneself, and actively use them to generate health. I think that my contact with native traditions, mainly their personal experiences of the soul and the existence of a higher power, played a major role in my learning how to do so and eventually conquering the disease.'

The discussion continued through the evening, containing queries that could well summarise the previous chapters in this book: could human consciousness align itself to universal harmony, is freedom individualised, do belonging and separatism affect our lives and, if so, in which way, and many others. We agreed that few are the situations in life in which such a direct threat is made to the core of one's existence as when health goes away and, with it, the valuable sense of control, vitality and independence. Anthony, like countless other human beings afflicted by illness, described a typical occurrence in which, while desperately searching for a solution, one finds oneself powerless, angry and disoriented, fearing the worst and incapable of preventing it.

Present limitations in some medical areas, such as cancer diagnosis and treatment, infectious diseases, psychosomatic and neurological disorders and others are understandably accepted with difficulty by our contemporaries who, much as Anthony, are accustomed to advanced medical facilities. Consequently, they become increasingly attracted to a more global medical approach, integrating various disciplines and healing traditions, although their methods may sometimes appear old-fashioned, 'non-scientific' and unreliable.

Clearly, technological improvements occurring in medicine over the last hundred years have been such that people, unfamiliar with the intricacies of biological sciences, have had some difficulty in following the increase in the number of new drugs and the appearance of a multitude of diagnostic and therapeutic modalities. The functioning of the latter remains generally out of bounds for the unacquainted, despite the current extensive popularisation of scientific matters in the media. People therefore have the feeling that, in the last instance, the control over their health lies in the hands of the treating physician, without much place left for personal patient input.

Recent medical advances, as a train that travels at great speed and successfully conquers immense distances, demand a degree of effort and dedication that does not leave enough space for individualised passenger attention. In other words, the modern physician, despite being the possessor of great theoretical and practical knowledge, as well as benefiting from the support of numerous technical improvements, continues to be faced with a difficult daily task. His or her usual schedule includes an ever-increasing number of patients requiring a multitude of investigations and treatments, plus scientific research work and administrative arrangements. In this context, inevitably, time and nature, the two great benefactors revered by ancient healers, are losing their decisive influence over the medical domain.

With a mixture of hope and anxiety there is currently much talk about the future. Recent recollections of ancient medical traditions seem to be the natural result of modern society's search for answers among the difficulties encountered in the prevention and management of numerous diseases. Notwithstanding the obvious superiority of modern medicine in the amassed scientific knowledge, a review of ancient healing practices can add a valuable dimension to modern medical care, by bringing back the forgotten sense of a profession practised with a strong connection with our natural habitat and the appreciation of a quieter, more relaxed pace of living and acting.

This insight may bring about inner changes in one's consciousness, opening new ways of contemplation, manipulation and enhanced healing capabilities. In Albert Einstein's archives, originally kept at Princeton University in the United States and now with the Hebrew University in Jerusalem, a poignant statement can be found: 'I admit thoughts influence the body.' Coming from a scientist of Einstein's stature, the conclusion is of paramount importance, demonstrating the continuation into the twentieth century of philosophical precepts already existing, as we have seen, in oldest antiquity.

An elaborate scheme of action seems to be seldom necessary. Basically, the elevation of human thought to a spiritual dimension of reality appears to constitute the core performance, able to set in motion the powerful engine of mental and corporeal restoration. In this context, our predecessors' world views and healing techniques point towards a comprehensive, poetic and cosmically unifying perspective in which the mind–body relationship is but one of its fascinating aspects.

Egyptian priests, Tibetan monks, ancient Greek physicians and Amerindian shamans all left a legacy of a therapeutical system at the basis of which stood the need for a radical change in the mental and emotional state of the treated individual. This was mainly grasped as an awareness of the need for development, an opening of 'inner gates', permitting the instillation of a new life rhythm, different from the one the patient was accustomed to. Representing a crucial momentum in the curing process, this process altered old habits and generated a chain reaction of beneficial adjustments, including tranquillity, confidence and optimism.

Human potential, strongly emphasised by this approach, resulted in the active participation of the sufferer in the healing process, while fully exploiting his or her, intuitive and creative capacities. Dreamwork and storytelling, as we have previously seen, became an inherent part of ancient healing techniques, aimed primarily at the discovery of one's subconscious motivations, and were added to a line of complicated rituals, signifying the indivisible connection of the human psyche with the eternal matrix of the universe.

Maintaining current health and preventing future illnesses went hand in hand with strengthening existent resources, in a unique and significant integration of all levels of one's being – physical, emotional, mental and social. Understanding this vital interrelation, and applying it to modern medical diagnosis and treatment, has significant chances of enriching and enlarging today's wide-ranging arsenal of approaches.

Despair about life, disappointment arising from unrealistic goals, a sense of isolation, and unsatisfying relationships are some of the main contributors to health problems. Most can be influenced by a change in mental perspective, including a view of human existence as a temporary manifestation of an infinite, all-comprehensive entity. In the final analysis, our ancestors' attitude towards illness and health reflects an overwhelming belief in the capacity of the human mind to connect to this entity and, in case of need, to draw from it the stamina for recovery.

On the brink of the new millennium, humanity will certainly review the fruits of its developed intellect, assessing *de novo* Man's place in our planet's natural chain of life. When ill health, a major disturbance in mankind's ability to function and survive is seen as suggestive of a more comprehensive malaise than just one expressed on the physical level, it is of great importance to learn from recent years' medical experience. The following chapters will do just that, while assessing modern tendencies and highlighting efficient ways of incorporating the lessons of the past into contemporary medical practices. Essentially, they will analyse the use of one's hidden and powerful mental and emotional energies into healing processes, which unceasingly reattach the individual to a benevolent, nurturing and immutable whole.

PART III

A MIND OF OUR OWN

Chapter 1

Mind Bridges: Scientific versus Folk Psychology

*Teach us delight in simple things,
And mirth that has no bitter spring;
Forgiveness free of evil done,
And love to all men 'neath the sun!*

Rudyard Kipling, 'The Children's Song'

Knowledge enhances life. It is often considered that the more you know, the better you can appreciate life's offerings and can develop the balancing abilities required to walk existence's tightrope. One may wonder, though, if reality confirms this supposition.

In the medical domain, attempting to analyse this means having to deal with health promotion and maintenance issues, including the continuous struggle against a never-ending series of illnesses. Concerned with these topics is the field of health psychology. This is a relatively new area of inquiry, as the concept of an individual's mental and emotional involvement in his or her body's functioning, although being of ancient origin as we have previously seen, has only recently become developed enough to have been offered the status of an independent discipline.

While covering such important concerns as health education, the study of specific behaviour patterns triggering certain diseases, health policy formation and many others, scientists researching these domains provide an important contribution to the shaping of a new contemporary perception, based on an inherent, self-regulatory biological system.

For a therapist, the prevention and management of illness presents a complex, ever-changing pattern which requires much adaptability and taking into consideration numerous contributing elements: environmental influences, dietary habits, genetic constitution, the presence of risk factors, and so on. Additionally, it is probably correct to assume that a certain antagonism exists between, on the one hand, rational medical appraisal, based on practical experience, comparative studies and accredited definitions and, on the other, the personal, intimate participation of a patient.

> We are the music makers,
> And we are the dreamers of dreams,
> Wondering by lone sea-breakers,
> And sitting by desolate streams;
> World-losers and world-forsakers,
> On whom the pale moon gleams:
> Yet we are the movers and shakers
> Of the world for ever, it seems.

Man's ironic self-rating in the face of life's enormous demands is accurately captured in this 'Ode' by the poet Arthur

O'Shaughnessy. Despite obvious human limitations, the central feeling is nevertheless that of people building their lives according to a powerful self-image. 'I'm here to stay; I can do what I want,' seems to be the message.

Disease and physical incapacitation are possibly the most serious agents infringing on such a statement and the important drive and confidence contained in it. Illness strikes at the core of one's body 'visualisation', stuns personal development and, in most cases, no amount of emotional maturity can sufficiently counteract its effects.

The question to be asked is, how can the gap be bridged? What are the ways in which a transformation can be made of innocence, simplicity and spontaneity, some of the most profound and valuable dimensions of human nature, to the well-organised, highly rational world of science? Or, put another way, how can the awesome machine of modern medicine be brought to refine its movements, embrace the individual in a serene, personalised care, and enhance the patient's own potential to fight illness?

For someone willing to conquer an acute or chronic disorder, or for a person interested in protecting and prolonging his or her well-being, the required fundamental process is the integration of mental, physical, emotional and spiritual resources in order to attain the desired goal. This comprehensive performance is not something that unfolds naturally at the push of a button, nor is it usually clearly contemplated by the person in need. Ego, the forcible master, employs innumerable subterfuges to conceal the meandering roads to the final truth. A change in consciousness is therefore called for, leading to the discovery of a wealth of inner resources and self-healing capabilities.

In this context, it is important to underline the significance of the malleability of the human mind, of its dynamism and modifiable mode of action, as opposed to the rigid nature of the body. Essentially, the mind becomes clay in the masterly hands of an ingenious psyche. As a result, to the normal imprint of a genetic matrix, completed by social and cultural marks, can be added useful and multiple amendments promoting a better life.

And how should these consciousness changes take place? A great body of literature has been dedicated to the subject in recent years, promoting various approaches, including meditation, physical exercise, dietary regimens, transpersonal psychotherapy, dream analysis, colour and aroma therapy, and many others. Already in 1983, A Sheikh, in *Imagery: Current Theory, Research and Applications* (Wiley) reported on a fall in blood pressure in patients using relaxation methods, which included slow breathing, as well as muscle and mental relaxation obtained by imagining pleasant experiences.

Since then, the number of medical reports on similar successes has grown significantly. They all underline the positive influence exerted on organic symptoms by reducing mental distress and anxiety. Nevertheless, it looks as though the huge growth in relaxation techniques remains beneficial only if the end result is the build-up of the patient's own problem-solving skills and his or her release from therapeutic dependency.

This goal appears to be one of the most difficult to attain. A possible path in this direction and towards forming an ideal programme of 'self-liberation' is the comprehension of the differences between the scientific approach to disease and a less rational, more inwardly attuned view. Practically speaking, successful coping with drastic changes in one's life requires a well-developed sense of self-reliance and independence. Clinical studies investigating the behaviour of patients with a variety of ailments can indeed show that under stressful circumstances the intensity of response is related to a patient's feeling of control.

This valid point can be supported by advising patients to 'go back to their roots', to their innate 'ideas' existing a priori in all human beings. Guy Claxton suggested in a recent book entitled *Hare Brain, Tortoise Mind* (Fourth Estate, 1998) that it is possible to become more 'intelligent' when thinking less, signifying 'putting to sleep' the conscious mind and letting the rich and knowledgeable subconscious take over and come up with the right answers.

Returning to essential, primordial human capabilities is a complex process. It has to do with the age-long controversy between Cartesian views, represented by notorious philosophers of the past such as René Descartes, Immanuel Kant and the contemporary linguist Noam Chomsky, and empirical ideas, similar to those expressed by the British philosophers John Locke and David Hume. The former maintained that certain ideas (for example those of self, God, time and inspiration) are innate, i.e. are 'preprinted' in the human mind, while the latter philosophers minimised the importance of inborn traits and underlined the great value of practical experience in the shaping of one's personality.

Popular traditions seem to align themselves with Descartes's rational doctrine. In a rich and extensive worldwide lore, numerous cultural heroes have always been depicted as resorting to their innermost powers when fighting evil. In the resulting liberation process, all wounds are healed and all wrongs made right, but not without due honour being accorded to persistence, flexibility, hope and audacity, essential ingredients for a positive outcome. From Prometheus to Coyote, and from Robin Hood to Yamato-takeru, all legends describe the accomplishments of admired heroes as a prototype of Man's struggle to overcome his inherent weaknesses and physical limitations.

If there are any lessons to be learned, they certainly pertain to causative factors in everyday life and human behaviour in particular circumstances. When afflicted by illness, it is advisable to review basic reasons for happiness and the amount of conformity and prejudice in one's life. 'A truly great man never puts away the simplicity of a child', says a Chinese proverb. The guiding line will be therefore to search for a primal innocence, a state of mind that eliminates the bias existing as a result of hard cultural assumptions.

The regained state of being will open a window through which it is easy to contemplate the other dimension of well-being, a form of existence in which certain self-imposed lines of thought and conduct permit one to achieve far-reaching results. 'Our life is frittered away by detail... Simplify, simplify,' advised the US writer Henry David Thoreau in *Walden, where I lived and what I lived for*. To this can be added: revise your priorities, take responsibility, perceive a crisis as a challenge or an opportunity for a change to something better, take action by considering options and make a decision based on your ability to handle problems and overcome adverse circumstances successfully.

'Getting better' becomes a programme of self-liberation, a journey that replaces one's feeling of being suspended by a thread over a raging sea with a solid raft to cling on to: one's own will and determination. Acts performed in simplicity and innocence are within anybody's reach, without any need for philosophical speculations. They start exactly where reason ends and can provide the required substratum for the expression of the unspoken, innate human potential, capable of resolving conflict, tolerating frustration and adapting to change.

There is vast empirical validation for the above, mainly from the field of behavioural medicine, which deals with interventions meant to train patients to alter the physiological conditions responsible for their problems. This is done by a process of strengthening and stabilisation, through reducing impatience, anger, irritation and hostility. These distracting emotions represent central obstacles in the creation of a favourable climate permitting coping and recovery. The deepening of one's awareness, self-acceptance and self-confidence, as a powerful mountain torrent, opens the way out of negative preconditioning and emotional confusion, while removing blocking debris of helplessness and self-deception invariably leading to failure.

In a recent book, *Worrying – Perspectives on Theory, Assessment and Treatment*, edited by Graham Davey and Frank Tallis (John Wiley & Sons, Chichester, 1994), the authors detail the central role played by pessimistic future beliefs together with an anxious mood, in forming negative judgement processes. When directed to focus on why an adverse outcome is likely, one finds it increasingly difficult to think of counter examples for that possibility. Worriers and non-worriers seem to differ not only in their reserves of knowledge, but in presenting a persistent pattern of recurring aversive thoughts and a continuous retrieval of previously contrary judgements.

Battling illness requires the type of intervention that would seriously reduce this negativity and facilitate a more positive thinking strategy, while musing on the successful alternative and the reasons for its happening. This is the environment of thought and feeling under which one can recruit coping resources to deal with the threatening situation effectively. It represents in many ways the subject of transpersonal therapy, which in recent times has attempted to combine conventional psychotherapy and scientific approaches with other disciplines related to personal growth and cognitive change, such as meditation, imagery and dream work, yoga, ecological interest, and others.

In *The Development of Personality* (Princeton University Press), the renowned Swiss psychoanalyst Carl Gustav Jung wrote, 'Fortunately, in her kindness and patience, Nature has never put the fatal question as to the meaning of their lives into the mouth of most people. And where no one asks, no one needs to answer.' A large portion of humanity lives its life without the capability or interest to dwell in the misty waters of the unconscious or to unravel the enigmas of God and the universe. Only when misfortune strikes are their beliefs and inner powers placed to the test. Only then are experience, background and education, cultural tradition, intuition of self-evident truths and logical deductions brought under one roof as a last resort in the pressing combat.

Most of the time the many obstacles in one's path constitute an entity that cannot entirely be grasped by the intellect. In order to reject despair and begin the process of healing, life has to be visualised not as a condition of static perfection, but as an ongoing process of change, a symptom of its infinity and submission to universal interconnection. In this context, there is place in modern medicine for free human deliberation, especially when accompanied by important traits: simplicity, spontaneity and serenity, as beneficial as they are age-long and elementary.

Chapter 2

Keeping the Faith – Spirituality and Healing

If one does not know to which port one is sailing, no wind is favourable.

Seneca

Over the centuries, Man's experience of reality and his moral precepts have carried the stigma of a powerful and as yet unresolved conflict. The battle between good and evil, as well as the painful dilemma of human mortality and suffering, clearly continuing to prevail in the world despite the supposed existence of a divine order, represents a permanent and agonising subject of preoccupation.

Pioneering philosophers, such as Aristotle and Plato, based the concept of polarity and striking dissimilarity between good and evil on the principles of the metaphysical dualism of matter and form. For their followers, and for anyone else attempting to comprehend the meaning of the inherent struggle in human existence, the ancient question of the origin of evil remains unanswered.

Most major world religions see as a most distressing acceptance the potential origin of disruption, pain and deterioration in the divine realm of activity and creation. Often visualised as sources of love, grace and charity, celestial forces are considered humanity's perpetual allies, guides and protectors. Endless mythological and devotional images and symbols were therefore included into the world lore, in order to demonstrate the vital and unequivocal role played by the belief in supernatural dominance and counsel.

A lengthy discussion of a specific notion, which Socrates designated 'the perfected nature of man', lies outside the focus of this book. Described by the famous thinker as 'the sun of the philosopher, his root and his branch', the imagery relates to the connection between the creative and preserving divine forces and human life. As a unique element belonging to each individual, and unceasingly accompanying one throughout life, it has been considered by ancient philosophers to represent the intellect of Man, his shadow and his benefactor, intrinsically connected both with a human being's unmatched essence and the surrounding universe.

The 'perfected nature of man', the angel and the demon within, able to teach and reply to questions, opens wide, gate after gate, the strenuous road to knowledge. One of the most intriguing philosophical queries relates to the existence of Mephistopheles, the devil to whom the legendary magician Faust sold his soul and which can be perceived as a manifestation of the wandering scholar's inner world, an intellectual guide and an integral component of his psychological makeup.

The inimitable nature of human existence makes healing an all-important means for maintaining the perfection of creation, of supporting and enhancing the harmonious blending of mankind into the natural world. Socrates also said: 'Know thyself'. In the above context, this advice focuses fundamentally on the recognition of the inner guide, the personal protective angel, capable of proposing solutions that may ordinarily be considered unrealistic. The end result contains unlimited possibilities.

Whether or not Man is capable of communicating with this inner oracle is an issue that has preoccupied philosophers and scientists continuously through the ages. In the midst of noticed cultural variations, many Eastern religious traditions promoted a higher degree of interiorisation in the devotional process and more personal involvement. Their central doctrines stress the importance of quiet contemplation and attunement with the highest forces of the universe, techniques able to create a sense of divine approachability and of immediate and tangible help available. The resulting state of being permits all inner human powers to be focused on the attainment of a proposed goal.

The recent popular embracing of Eastern philosophy and religion has made these methods available throughout the world and in many ways instigated a renewed exploration of the psycho-religious dynamics of consciousness, as well as of the powerful interaction of religious beliefs with the healing process. Dr Herbert Benson, of Harvard Medical School in the United States, has studied intensively the effects of faith and regular prayer on both the process of adaptability to disease, as well as the recovery from it, and has attempted to quantify such effects in various patients. Other researchers have done similar work at various medical centres throughout the world, focusing on health and spirituality and pondering on how the two may interact.

An interesting current trend, developing particularly in the US, is the introduction into the medical studies curriculum of programmes dealing with Eastern and Western religious traditions, as well as contemporary research covering different traditional healing practices. The main objective of these projects is to prepare physicians to better understand and range themselves with their patients' needs. Thus the scope of medical teaching is expanded with lectures on comparative religion, faith healing, native practices, herbal medicine, meditative techniques, biofeedback, and many others.

The prevailing perception is that nowadays medical practitioners should go beyond their traditional academic training and explore the role of the mind and spiritual beliefs on treatment outcome and the recovery process. In a recent article, 'Types of spiritual well-being among persons with chronic illness: their relation to various forms of quality of life', published in the *Archives of Physical Medicine and Rehabilitation*, Dr Barth Riley and colleagues reported on types of spiritual well-being among persons with chronic illness and their relation to various forms of quality of life. Selecting 216 chronic inpatients at a US midwestern medical centre, the authors classified them accordingly to their spiritual beliefs in religious, existential and nonspiritual.

The results of the study showed that subtypes differed significantly with respect to various aspects of quality of life. Moreover, they demonstrated that, compared with other cluster groups, the nonspiritual group reported significantly lower levels of quality of life and life satisfaction, and the highest proportion of health-status change with respect to both improvement and decline in health.

Additionally, Harold Koenig, a psychiatrist from Duke University in the US, in 1996 released a study, based on 4,000 randomly selected people, which showed that older people who attend religious services are physically healthier, less anxious and feel less isolated and helpless. The authors of both studies agree that further consistent and peer-reviewed research is needed to validate their results. They join nevertheless the increasing efforts of numerous scientists, physicians, psychologists, sociologists and theologians who are currently attempting to define the exact role that devotional prayer may play in combating disease and disability.

It is therefore not surprising that an editorial published in 1998 in the highly respected *Journal of the American Medical Association* (JAMA) (Mar., 79: 258–64) called for manuscripts to be sent in dealing with complementary therapies considered fit to be integrated into clinical practice. The article encouraged the performance of high-quality, randomised clinical trials, in order to evaluate 'the efficacy, safety, outcomes, and cost-effectiveness of complementary and alternative medical interventions.'

Among the new suggested techniques, patients' spiritual beliefs occupy a special place. Their introduction has to overcome the known historical rift between scientific medicine and religious doctrines, the fierce antagonism arising from the legitimate attempt of dedicated researchers to protect themselves and their discoveries from the dark shadows of ignorance and superstition. On the other hand, theologians have often faced increasing pressure from scientific atheism, which continuously excluded the need to determine the place or actions of a ruling God, and tended to present nature as a self-sufficient mechanism.

Notwithstanding, a major international news magazine (*Newsweek*, 27 July, 1998) proclaimed recently that 'Science found God', enthusiastically describing the increasing ability of scientific research and religious doctrines to cooperate in their pursuit for the eternal and unique truth. As part of this tantalising process, modern times have seen a re-enactment of discussions on mind–body interaction, i.e. on the ways in which, either through relaxation-induced responses or positive thinking, the human intellect and psychological makeup can influence physical health. This inevitably touched such areas as the curing power of time, the importance of healing relationships, and the value of ceremony and ritual in strengthening one's belief in success.

All the above notions, commonly found in major religious teachings and with native holistic healers, supplement the idea of creating an integrative medical approach, expected to enhance patients' own defence capabilities, reduce hospital stays and improve general life quality. While reconsidering the highly beneficial cooperation between medicine and major spiritual traditions of the world, room is created for more personal involvement in the healing process, with a patient being offered the possibility to 'work at it', 'stop commiserating' and learn how, amidst numerous experts and while taking advice, to find his or her own way and maintain the all-important personal power and confidence.

Modern religious beliefs attempt to eliminate the need to view disease as a punishment and hope to be able to guide a patient towards purity, knowledge, understanding and inner peace. In the manner viewed by ancient philosophers, humanity, in desperate need to conquer illness and suffering, is offered the chance to rediscover the light of the spiritual flow. Originating from the highs of the intellect, it gloriously shines through, penetrates the 'material' body and is able to assist medical treatment in achieving its full effect.

Chapter 3

Acting on Instinct and the Twists of Reason

A moment's insight is sometimes worth a life's experience.

Oliver Wendell Holmes,
The Professor at the Breakfast Table

Of all the issues relating to self-transformation, none is so fitting as the metamorphosis of abstract concepts and visual ideas into concrete results. In order to achieve that, the human mind needs to balance and reconcile not only knowledge, experience and observation, but also the capability of inner awareness, or perception by intuition. In the light of this faculty, numerous phenomena marking one's life may hold a special and intriguing significance.

Apart from its classical definition of 'direct perception without conscious attention or reasoning', intuition has a spiritual connotation and has been likened to a sixth sense. It can explain gut feeling, the ability to 'just know' something, the danger sense, unexpected luck, and the drawing of immediate conclusions without rational or logical inference. Intuition can mean 'hold on to your dreams', 'let's call him up', 'go to the right', 'I'm leaving', 'I'm staying', and innumerable other instantaneous decisions and revelations, springing from one's deepest mental recesses. It never offers explanations, but just points towards the right direction, in a moment of grace, often in the midst of momentous turmoil.

Viewed essentially as a search for the most suitable path to follow for the ultimate truth, intuition is traditionally compared to reasoning. In the frame of one's attempt to preserve health or cure illness, the closest notion that comes to mind is that of moral reasoning (promoted by Aristotle), which emphasises the quest for the best means of attaining the highest moral good. Aristotle identified this entity with happiness, considered by him as a primordial goal to be pursued by all of humanity.

Various virtues, such as courage and determination, may support one in achieving this end. Reason will thus propose actions needed to be performed in order to be courageous and determined. This capability has been named practical reasoning, since in this manner reason guides human acts. Cold and sterile as it may seem, reasoning denotes an important process of forming arguments and drawing 'logical' conclusions, and forms an integral and crucial part of scientific work and deduction.

At the same time, there are recurring cases recorded in the history of science when a sudden insight or a unique clarifying idea springs into the consciousness of a researcher and revolutionises the existent knowledge, without having recourse to logical inquiry. Such products of scientific intuition demonstrate that both sudden inspiration and reasoning do not occur in isolation, but as a combined tool for achieving progress.

All things considered, intuition may not always offer a final solution, but it certainly opens new directions for thought and accomplishment. To this must be added the fact that Aristotle's view, concerning the best ways to attain the highest ethical good, has been often criticised, as it is improbable that such a unique, well-defined entity exists. In fact, hopes and ideals are as individual as people are, and therefore the significance of intuitive human powers, used in combination with the logic of analysis, lies mainly in the practical results to which individuals may arrive by employing them.

And what are the possible consequences of one's ability to not only perceive basic truths rationally, but also to cultivate intuition as a source of new vitality, as well as a problem-solving and decision-making tool? Some points would include:

* Making a sound judgement to guide action.
* Integrating a number of factors and proposing a speedy and appropriate solution.
* Coping with partial information and building upon it complete and satisfactory results.
* Deciding correctly on the acceptance or rejection of an opportunity.
* Recognising motivations and intentions in other people.
* Developing a sense of 'aliveness' and creativity as a result of positive performances.
* Achieving emotional balance and spiritual awareness.

In an article entitled 'The paradox of the rational patient and the ethical physician' (appearing as part of the Internet Journal *Mathematical Issues of Scientific Medicine* in 1997), Michael F Quinn, of the Emory University School of Medicine in Atlanta, discusses the struggle for an optimal diagnostic process; presenting the issue as a formal mathematical problem, Dr Quinn considers that 'no physician or algorithm, however good, can make decisions that guarantee the best possible outcome to every patient. A patient faces a medical lottery created by nature and exhibits rational decision-making behaviour by minimising personal risk. In contrast, one physician is personally accountable for medical decisions made on behalf of many patients and assumes the ethical responsibility of a lottery administrator to allocate risk equitably and impartially.'

While doctor and patient can be seen as pursuing identical goals, their cooperation and personal interaction are subject to a great variety of constraints, which add to the complexity of the medical decision-making process and leave the door wide open for supportive circumstances. Among them, the reinforcement of the intuitive capabilities of both the physician and the patient seem to play an important role.

Sigmund Freud is known to have written: 'When making a decision of *minor* importance, I have always found it advantageous to consider all the pros and cons. In *vital* matters, however, such as the choice of a mate or a profession, the decision should come from the unconscious. The important decisions of our personal life should be governed by the deep inner needs of our nature.' Health problems can undoubtedly be added to this.

In recent years, medical literature has demonstrated a continuous preoccupation with growing a patient's involvement in the diagnostic and therapeutic processes. Mentioning but a few titles could well exemplify this trend: Kasper, J, Mulley, A and Wennberg, J, 'Developing shared decision-making programs to improve the quality of health care' (*Quality Review Bulletin*, vol. 18, June 1992); Deber, RB, 'Shared decision-making in the real world' (*Journal of General Internal Medicine*, vol. 11, June 1996); Kennedy, M, 'Making patients part of their healthcare team' (*The Quality Letter for Healthcare Leaders*, vol. 7, no. 2, March 1995), and many others.

But how does one develop his or her intuitive faculties? Great social and emotional pressure accompanies most life events and, therefore, much conscious 'fog' is created by preconceived ideas, labels and emotions, often obscuring the richness, subtlety and power of unconscious advice. In the absence of the necessary knowledge and experience, like in many other fields of specialised expertise, the medical domain implies in the great majority of cases an almost exclusive usage of the doctor's decision on the main diagnosis and the treatment to be followed, as well as in signalling a recovery.

Learning to participate actively in the healing process means acquiring new skills or developing a new outlook in order to cope better with a stressful situation. There are many stumbling blocks to this initiation, including anxiety, negativity, previous unsatisfactory experiences, inflexibility and low self-esteem. In order to deal with them, a complete change in attitude is necessary, the complexity of which is enhanced by the fact that intuition is a spontaneous occurrence that cannot be programmed in advance.

On one hand, the establishment of a specific plan for the accomplishment of one's goals can prove considerably efficient. It may be of great help to state: 'I want to get better and this is what I'm going to do in order to achieve this objective.' Carefully weighing the alternatives may prove initially frightening, but may provide an unexpected source of encouragement and determination, as natural human resilience and love of life will generally direct one towards battling illness forcefully.

Unfortunately, outlining a project may interfere with the characteristics of the intuitive hunch. Still, while aims are well delineated, one can create the conditions under which a healthy and powerful insight may become active. Here again, some valuable rules may be identified:

* Approach a problem with great flexibility.
* Search for an atmosphere of serenity and mental relaxation. Numerous solutions to troubling issues become apparent when walking in the freshness of a beautiful park or strolling on the beach, while taking a bath or a shower, or when listening to inspirational music.
* Do not struggle to find an instantaneous answer to a problem. Time is a great adviser. So is sleep.
* Free yourself from old thinking patterns. Let your mind run wild and your senses awaken. Do not discard any idea as too 'irrational' to be taken into consideration.
* Visualise illness as a process of self-transformation, an eye-opener and an important challenge. While doing so, stand back and await for your inner guidance to surprise you by its astoundingly appropriate advice.

People may be certainly discouraged by discovering the amount of self-reliance and hard work required in order to use these guidelines. Permanent mental and physical health are rarely a gift. Their maintenance is inevitably accompanied by a veritable test of endurance, including the necessity of remaining focused, positive and constructive at all times. How many among us can pride ourselves of being capable to do so?

The problem becomes more acute at the time of a health crisis, when specific ideas and plans have to be found in order to ensure an eventual success. In most cases, a complete remake of one's attitude towards healing and one's defence capabilities will serve as the decisive factor in the recovery effort. Sacrifices are often necessary.

Renouncing old habits such as smoking, consumption of alcohol and coffee, or overeating, well entrenched in a person's life and clearly detrimental, may represent powerful compensatory elements and recognised security blankets difficult to give up.

Moreover, in health matters, it is surprising how difficult it appears to leave dependency – the viewpoint that somebody else can decide for you – even for people with active professional lives, accustomed to making decisions. One of my patients, a successful bank manager, was suffering from thyrotoxicosis, a hyperactive state of the thyroid gland. Drug therapy, well developed and recognised in this disorder, did not succeed in alleviating classical complaints such as rapid heart beat, insomnia, irritability and agitation. We soon realised that changing medical therapy would not be of help. What the young woman needed was a total change in lifestyle and behaviour patterns, achievable through a relaxation programme.

A main hindrance in attempts to participate actively in one's own healing process is to immediately assume the worst and decide that 'I wish I could help, but it is too late to change.' Much like medical students who tend to think they suffer from every illness in the textbook, people nowadays, due to the large amount of medical data available, create their own images as to the seriousness of their medical condition and the possible ways to approach it. Very often, misinformation results in making major decisions in a highly emotional state, significantly impairing the quality of the judgement.

Many people perceive taking a stand and preparing to fight illness as being the actions of an unrealistic idealist, uselessly attempting to change direction and restructure a life pattern, at the most inappropriate time, when one's inner powers appear to be at their lowest. Paradoxically, one of the contributing reasons to this attitude is the information the patient receives on his or her condition. While carrying obvious legal and ethical implications, the sombre, dry tone with which these explanations are often being offered brings about an immediate suppression of the patient's natural optimism and creativity.

'It is easier to move a mountain, than change one's personality,' says a Chinese proverb. In order to succeed, it seems that there is a need for both the physician and the patient to adopt a similar attitude, one that permanently excludes the 'business as usual' approach. As difficult as it may be to stay empathic, centred and unhesitating at all times, medical treatment should be able to not only end in a cure, but also offer a generalised improvement, capable of providing lifelong protection against disease.

The much talked-about self-healing potential has a great deal to do with what was named in recent years 'psychoneuroimmunology', i.e. the study of the immune reactions occurring in the human body as a result of changes in the psychological state of an individual. Based on extensive research, scientists around the world have begun to identify an intimate connection between one's emotional makeup and responsiveness to illness. In view of the crucial role played by the immune system in the susceptibility to disease, as well as in the ability of one's body to fight lethal cells and toxic substances, the importance of such studies cannot be underestimated.

In view of this, Hippocrates's saying: 'Tell me who you are and I will tell you what kind of disease you may develop' acquires its entire relevance. Not only does mental discipline promote a harmonious interaction with one's environment, but it may eliminate unnecessary fear, anger, worry and sadness, all powerful inner antagonists to successful medical care.

Being relaxed, friendly and optimistic, as well as expressing your emotions outwardly and honestly, may, according to recent evidence that fully supports Hippocrates's ancient view, ensure better health.

Apart from genetic, nutritional and environmental factors, the mind–body interplay represents a vital component in the appearance of numerous diseases. This intriguing channel, when activated in the right manner, is able to dissipate the thick smokescreen concealing the self-generated, beneficial healing powers of an individual. By using these powers, as opposed to feeling frail, self-conscious and disoriented, a patient may respond to illness with a positive, stable and courageous attitude, which will boost the immune system and increase the chances of victory against disease.

As inconceivable as it seems, the power to manipulate cell functioning and metabolism through the power of one's thoughts is an authentic and integral component of a whole system of self-protection designed to bypass emotional responses such as denial, anxiety or depression. In cases of acute or chronic illness, behavioural and cognitive interventions, such as biofeedback, diversion and restructuring, as well as insight and family therapy, are all aimed at strengthening the above system and releasing its full benefits as a successful adaptive mean.

Nevertheless, assistance from trained professionals can be substantially enhanced by personal contributions. It is in everyone's capability to access this 'fountain of inner wisdom', when imagery and meditation are some of the main approaches used for this purpose. 'I have stilled and quieted my soul like a weaned child with his mother' (Psalms 13:12). Quieting one's mind may mean eliminating interference from one's thoughts or, as Einstein said, 'the multitude of things that clutter up the mind and divert it from the essentials'. This will invariably allow core issues and intuitive ideas to come to the forefront.

'All great ... achievements,' Einstein also considered, 'start from intuitive knowledge, namely, in axioms, from which deductions are then made... Intuition is the necessary condition for the discovery of such axioms.' In the turmoil and imbalance created by disease, being capable of registering the 'axioms', i.e. the self-evident truths, the insightful directives for one's subconscious mind, appears to be, for both the physician and the patient, as deeply significant and as instrumental as it is in the work of a dedicated researcher. That the mind can heal is no longer a speculative folklore, but a distinct possibility.

Bibliography

Books

Achterberg, J: *Imagery in Healing*, Shambhala, 1985
Amundsen, DW: *Medicine, Society and Faith in the Ancient and Medieval Worlds*, Johns Hopkin University Press, 1996
Aristotle (transl. Rackham, H): *The Nichomachean Ethics*, Harvard University Press, 1982
— (ed. Ross, WD and Ross, D): *Aristotelis Analytica Priora et Posteriora*, Clarendon Press, 1981
Armstrong, DM: *The Nature of Mind*, Cornell University Press, 1980

Bateson, G: *Mind and Nature: A Necessary Unit*, Bantam, 1998
Benson, H: *The Relaxation Response*, Morrow, 1975
Bergson, H: *The Creative Mind – An Introduction to Metaphysics*, Citadel Press, 1997
— (transl. Palmer, WS and Paul, NM): *Matter and Memory*, Zone Books, 1991

Bodde, D: *A Short History of Chinese Philosophy*, The Free Press, 1976

Byrne, PH: *Analysis and Science in Aristotle*, State University of New York Press, 1997

Calvin, WH: *How Brains Think – Evolving Intelligence Then and Now*, Weidenfeld & Nicolson, 1996

Cassidy, D: *Einstein and Our World*, Humanities Press, 1995

Chomsky, N: *Language and Mind*, Harcourt Brace Jovanovich, 1972

— *Language and the Problems of Knowledge*, MIT Press, 1980

Churchland, PM: *Matter and Consciousness*, Bradford Books, MIT Press, 1984

Cohen, MN: *Health and the Rise of Civilization*, Yale University Press, 1989

Cooper, C (ed.): *Handbook of Stress, Medicine and Health*, CRC Press, 1996

Copeland, J: *Artificial Intelligence – a Philosophical Introduction*, Blackwell Publishers, 1993

Cousins, N: *Human Options*, WW Norton & Co, 1981

Crick, F: *The Astonishing Hypothesis – The Scientific Search for the Soul*, Touchstone, 1994

Dalley, S: *Myths from Mesopotamia*, Oxford University Press, 1989

Dawson, C: *Matthew Arnold: The Poetry (The Collected Critical Heritage: Victorian Thinkers)*, Routlege, 1995

Dennett, DC: *Kinds of Minds*, Weidenfeld & Nicolson, 1996

Descartes, R (ed. Cottingham, J and Williams, B): *Meditations on First Philosophy: with Selections from the Objections and Replies*, Cambridge University Press, 1996

Dohrenwend, BS and Dohrenwend, BP: *Stressful Life*

Bibliography

Events: Their Nature and Effects, John Wiley and Sons, 1974

Dossey, L: *Space, Time and Medicine*, New Science Library, Boston, 1982

Dumont, L: *Religion, Politics and History in India*, Mouton Publishers, Paris, 1970

Einstein, A: *The World as I See It*, Citadel Press, 1931
— *Ideas and Opinions*, Crown, 1954
— *Out of my later years: The scientist, philosopher and man portrayed through his own words*, Outlet, 1993

Eysenck, M: *Attention and Arousal: Cognition and Performance*, Springer, 1990

Fagan, BM: *People of the Earth*, HarperCollins, 1995

Fideler, DR (ed.): *The Pythagorean Sourcebook and Library*, Phanes Press, 1987

Finger, S: *Origins of Neuroscience: A History of Explorations into Brain Function*, Oxford University Press, 1994

Frank AW: *The Wonderful Storyteller: Body, Illness and Ethics*, University of Chicago Press, 1995

Frank, J: *Persuasion and Healing*, Johns Hopkin University Press, 1974

Freud, S: *The Interpretation of Dreams*, Random House, 1978
— (transl. and ed. Strachey J: *The Complete Psychological Works of Sigmund Freud*, The Hogarth Press, 1966–74

Furnham, A: *All in the Mind – The Essence of Psychology*, Whurr Publishers, 1996

Galen: *On the Natural Faculties*, Harvard University Press, 1916

Gazzaniga, MS: *The Social Brain: Discovering the Networks of the Mind*, Basic Books, 1985

Guyton, HC: *Human Physiology and Mechanisms of Disease*, WB Saunders, 1982

Hawking, S: *A Brief History of Time*, Bantam Doubleday Dell, 1998

Herodotus: *The Histories*, Penguin, 1996

Hobson, JA: *The Chemistry of Conscious States: How the Brain Changes Its Mind*, Little, Brown, 1994

Holmes, OW, *The essential Holmes: Selections from letters, speeches, judicial opinions and other writings*, University of Chicago Press, 1996

Jackendoff, R: *Patterns in the Mind: Language and Human Nature*, Basic Books, 1994

Jeans, JH, *The Mysterious Universe*, AMS Press, 1933

Jung, CG: *Memories, Dreams, Reflections*, Vintage, 1961

Khalfa, J (ed.): *What is Intelligence?*, Cambridge University Press, 1994

Klein, M and Money-Kirle, RE: *Love, Guilt and Reparation and Other Works, 1921–45*, Free Press, 1984

Kovacs MG: *The Epic of Gilgamesh*, Stanford University Press, 1989

Landy, D (ed.): *Culture, Disease and Healing: Studies in Medical Anthropology*, Macmillan, 1997

La Mettrie, JO de: *Man a Machine*, Open Court, 1912

Lao Tzu: *Tao Te Ching – An Illustrated Journey*, Little, Brown 1994

Last, CG (ed.): *Anxiety Across the Lifespan: A Developmental Perspective*, Springer, 1993

Lawrence, DH: *Complete Poems* (Penguin Twentieth-Centurty Classics), Penguin, 1994

Bibliography

Leder, D (ed): *The Body in Medical Thought and Practice*, Kluwer Academic, 1995

Le Shan, L: *The Medium, the Mystic, and the Physicist*, Baltimore Books, 1975

Ling, T: *A History of Religion East and West*, Macmillan Press, 1968

McKeown, T: *The Origins of Human Diseases*, Blackwell Publishers, 1988

McGovern, A: *Aesop's Fables*, Scholastic Paperbacks, 1963

Meichenbaum, D and Jarenko, ME: *Stress Reduction and Prevention*, Plenum Press, 1983

Minsky, M: *The Society of Mind*, Simon & Schuster, 1986

Mithen, S: *The Prehistory of the Mind*, Thames & Hudson, 1997

Omstein, R: *The Psychology of Consciousness*, Arkana, Penguin, 1972

Palos, S: *The Chinese Art of Healing*, Herder & Herder, 1971

Peat, DF: *Synchronicity: The Bridge Between Mind and Matter*, Bantam Books, 1987

Penrose, R: *Shadows of the Mind – A Search for the Missing Science of Consciousness*, Vintage, 1994

Phillips, ED: *Greek Medicine*, Thames & Hudson, 1973

Pickering, J and Skinner, M: *From Sentence to Symbols – Readings on Consciousness*, Harvester Wheatsheaf, 1990

Pitcher, G: *Wittgenstein: The Phillosophical Investigations*, Doubleday, 1996

Pitts, M and Phillips, K (ed.): *The Psychology of Health*, Routledge, 1991

Plank, M: *Where is Science Going?*, Norton, 1932

Plato (ed. Cooper JM and Hutchinson DS): *Complete Works*, Hackett Pub. Co., 1997

Pylyshyn, ZW: *Computation and Cognition*, MIT Press, 1984

Richards, RJ *Darwin and the Emergence of Evolutionary Theories of Mind and Behaviour*, University of Chicago Press, 1987

Rosenthal, DM: *The Nature of Mind*, Oxford University Press, 1991

Russell, B: *The Analysis of Mind*, George Allen & Unwin, 1921

Rutter, M Tizard, J and Whitmore, K: *Education, Health and Behaviour*, Longmans, Green and Co, 1970

Schiller, F: *Paul Broca – Founder of French Anthropology, Explorer of the Brain*, Oxford University Press, 1992

Schoemaker, S: *Self-knowledge and Self-identity*, Cornell University Press, 1963

Searle, JR: *Minds, Brains and Science*, Harvard University Press, 1984

Shapiro, AK and Shapiro, E: *The Powerful Placebo: from Ancient Preist to Modern Physician*, The Johns Hopkin University Press, 1998

Sigerist, HE: *A History of Medicine*, Oxford University Press, 1961

Singer, JS and Pope, KS: *The Power of the Human Imagination*, Plenum, 1978

Snapper, J: *Chinese Lessons to Western Medicine*, Grune & Stratton, 1965

Spinoza, B (transl. Britan, HH): *The Principles of Cartesian Philosophy and the Metaphysical Thoughts*, Open Court Publishers, 1974

Bibliography

— (transl. Elwes, RHM): *Ethics*, Dover Publications, 1955
Sperber, D: *Experiencing Culture – A Naturalistic Approach*, Blackwell Publishers, 1996
Strachey, J: *The Complete Psychological Works of Sigmund Freud*, vol. 24, Hogarth Press, 1966–74

Tallis, F: *How to Stop Worrying*, Sheldon Press, 1990
Taton, R (ed.): *Ancient and Medieval Science from the Beginning to 1450*, Basic Books, 1963
Thoreau, HD: *Walden*, Princeton University Press, 1989
Thorwald, J: *Science and Secrets of Early Medicine*, Harcourt, Brace & World, 1963

Walsh, R and Vaughan, F (ed.): *Paths Beyond Ego*, GP Putnam's Sons, 1993
Warnock, M: *Imagination and Time*, Blackwell Publishers, 1994
Whybrow, PC: *A Mood Apart: a Thinker's Guide to Emotion and Its Disorders*, Picador, 1998
Wittgenstein, L (trans. Anscombe, GEM): *Philosophical Investigations*, Prentice Hall, 1973
Wollheim, R: *The Thread of Life*, Harvard University Press, 1984
Wolpe, J: *The Practice of Behaviour Therapy*, Pergamon, 1969
Wordsworth, W: *Selected Poetry*, Oxford University Press, 1998

Articles

Astin, JA: 'Stress reduction through mindfulness meditation. Effects on psychological symptomatology, sense of control, and spiritual experiences,' *Psychotherapy & Psychosomatics*, 66(2):97–106, 1997

Chiarmonte, DR: 'Mind–body therapies for primary care physicians,' *Primary Care Clinics in Office Practice*, 24(4): 787–807, 1997

Drury, BL: 'Alternative therapies for postoperative pain,' *Nursing Spectrum*, 7(17):20, 1997

Dwairy, M: 'A biopsychosocial model of metaphor therapy with holistic cultures,' *Clinical Psychology Review*, 17(7):719–32, 1997

Ermalinski, R, Hanson, PG, et al: 'Impact of body–mind treatment component on alcoholic inpatients,' *Journal of Psychological Nursing*, 35(7):39–45, 1997

Farquhar, J: 'Chinese medicine and the life of the mind. Are brains necessary?' *North Carolina Medical Journal*, 59(3): 188–90, 1998

Feldman, HA., McKinlay, JB, Potter, DA, et al: 'Nonmedical influences on medical decision making: an experimental technique using videotapes, factorial design, and survey sampling,' *Health Services Research*, vol. 23, nr. 3, 1997

Field, TM: 'Massage therapy effects,' *American Psychologist*, 53(12):1,270–81, 1998

Giedt, JF: 'Guided imagery. A psychoneuroimmunological intervention in holistic nursing practice,' *Journal of Holistic Nursing*, 15(2):112–127

Goodman, A: 'Organic unit theory: an integrative mind–body theory for psychiatry,' *Theoretical Medicine*, 18(4):357–78, 1997

Kern, D and Baker, J: 'A comparison of mind/body approach versus a conventional approach to aerobic dance,' *Women's Health Issues*, 7(1):30–7, 1997

Koening, HG: *The influence of religiosity, family-of-origin and self-efficacy on depression in older adults*, Journal of Religious Gerentology, vol. 9, nr. 4, 1996

La Forge, R: 'Mind–body fitness: encouraging prospects for

primary and secondary prevention,' *Journal of Cardiovascular Nursing*, 11(3):53–965,1997

Lis-Balchin, M: 'Essential oils and aromatherapy: their modern role in healing,' *Journal of the Royal Society of Health*, 117(5):324–9, 1997

Mayr, B and Mayr A: 'Interactions between the immune system and the psyche,' *Tierarztliche Praxis*. Ausgabet K Kleintiere/
heimtiere, 26(4):230–5, 1998

Meymandi, A: 'Brain and behaviour,' *North Carolina Medical Journal*, US, 59(3):181, 1998

Miller, T: The value of imagery in perioperative nursing,' *Seminars in Perioperative Nursing*, 7(2): 1089–13, 1998

Noonan, SS: 'Pain management. The mind matters,' *New Jersey Medicine*. 96(1):37–9, 1999

Popova, EI, Mikheev VF, *et al*: 'Functional rearrangements in the human brain during emotional self-regulation with biological feedback,' *Neuroscience & Behavioural Physiology*, 28 (1):8–16, 1998

Sawyer, J: 'The first Reiki practitioner in our operating room,' *AORN Journal*, 67(3):674–7, 1998

Schotanus, WM: Healthy ageing: the body/mind/spirit connection,' *Journal of the Medical Association of Georgia*, 86(2):127–8, 1997

Seers, K and Carroll, D: 'Relaxation techniques for acute pain management: a systematic review,' *Journal of Advanced Nursing*, 27(3):466–75, 1998

Silverstaein, B: 'A follow-up note on Freud 's mind-body dualism: what Ferenczi learned from Freud,' *Psychological Reports*. 80(2):369–70, 1997

Sloman, A: 'The emperor's real mind: review of Roger Penrose's "The Emperor's New Mind": concerning computers, minds and the laws of physics', *Artificial Intelligence*, 56(2–3), 1992

Taubes, T: 'Healthy avenues of the mind: psychological theory building and the influence of religion during the era of moral treatment,' *American Journal of Psychiatry*, 155(8): 1,001–8, 1988

Tweed, TA: 'Religion and healing. Cultivating a respectful ambivalence,' North Carolina *Medical Journal*, 59(3): 186–7, 1998

Van der Feltz-Cornelis, CM and Van Dyck, R: 'The notion of somatization: an artefact of the conceptualization of body and mind,' *Psychotherapy & Psychosomatics*, 66(3): 117–27, 1997

Van Dixhorn, J: 'Cardiorespiratory effects of breathing and relaxation instruction in myocardial infarction patients,' *Biological Psychology*, 49(1–2):123–35, 1998

Wijma, K, Melin, A, *et al*: 'Treatment of menopausal symptoms with applied relaxation: a pilot study,' *Journal of Behavioural Therapy & Experimental Psychiatry*, 28(4): 251–61, 1997

Williams, RB: 'The mind, the body, health, and disease. What do we know, what should we do?' *North Carolina Medical Journal*, 59(3):172–4, 1998

Witten, E: 'Duality, spacetime and quantum mechanics,' *Physics Today*, vol. 50, nr. 5, 1997